ETHNOVETERINARY MEDICINES USED PETS IN BRITISH COLUMBIA

Cheryl Lans, PhD

Vancouver, BC

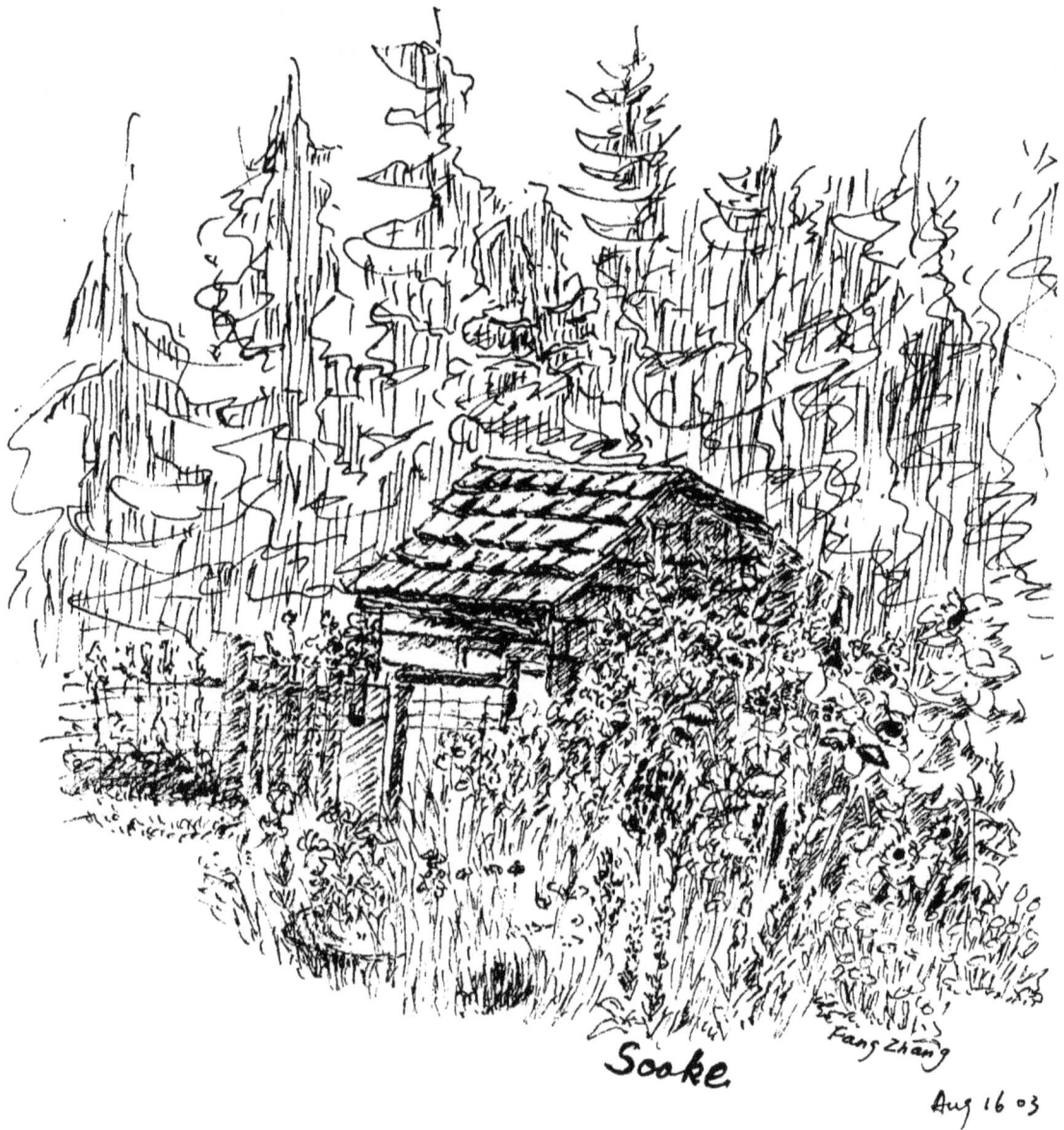

Sooke

Fang Zhang

Aug 16 03

Publisher: Lans, Cheryl 2012

ISBN: 978-0-9783468-9-8

Ethnoveterinary medicines used for pets in British Columbia 1

The research documented and validated (in a non-experimental way) the ethnoveterinary medicines used by livestock farmers and animal caretakers in British Columbia. The research was designed to contribute to farm incomes, maintain the resilience of farm communities, promote self-reliance and contribute to an internationally recognized safe and good quality food supply. It can also strengthen rural community capacity building, leadership and skills development.

Ethnoveterinary medicine is the scientific term for traditional animal health care. The use of medicinal plants, including to treat animals (ethnoveterinary medicine) is thousands of years old. Many non-Western traditions of veterinary medicine exist, such as acupuncture and herbal medicine in China, Ayurveda in India, etc. These traditions have written records that go back thousands of years (Hadani and Shimshony, 1994). Ethnoveterinary alternatives (based on medicinal plants) are necessary for small-scale livestock farmers and animal caretakers who cannot use allopathic drugs or for those larger conventional farmers whose economic circumstances prevent the use of veterinary services for minor health problems of livestock.

This research on ethnoveterinary remedies used in British Columbia addressed the question of how institutions can organize to bring about community-based technological solutions to participants' animal health problems based on traditional knowledge. In the context of this research on British Columbia (a resource-based economy), social resilience is the ability of farm communities to withstand external shocks (social, economic, political) and stresses like livestock diseases and illnesses. Ethnoveterinary medicines can be considered a form of *cultural capital*, which can stimulate livestock production or at minimum provide economic alternatives to allopathic drugs. *Social resilience* is a relevant concept since 7,460 farmers in British Columbia with annual sales of over $10,000 have a low net farm income. The return to assets on these farms ranges from –1% for farmers with sales of $19,000 to $25,000 to 5.2% from farms with sales of over $250,000. These figures are important because sustainable agriculture has been defined (by the Federal-Provincial Agriculture Committee on Environmental Sustainability) as that which is economically viable for the present generation of farmers and environmentally sustainable for the future generation.

The research also tested the potential of participatory workshops as a dissemination activity or new way of transferring knowledge in ethnoveterinary medicine. The International Institute of Rural Reconstruction (IIRR) developed the workshop method and it is said to have two major advantages; it reduces the total amount of time needed to develop information materials and it profits from the expertise and resources of a wide range of participants and their organizations. The workshop process results in the selection of ethnoveterinary practices and remedies that can be recommended for use by the general public and farmers to alleviate minor diseases and problems. The success of the ethnoveterinary project is partly based on the extent to which farmers and animal caretakers can use the resulting manual for improved livestock health; although it was not designed to replace standard veterinary information.

The second aspect to the success of this research is its acceptance by the scientific community. Five papers were published; one of these in a high-ranking veterinary journal Veterinary Parasitology. This book presents the unpublished research on ethnoveterinary medicines in pets. All of the treatments in the manual and those in this book are those that were deemed to be effective in either curing the problem or prolonging the pet's life.

The treatments for one raccoon are included in the results. These treatments are important because they took place over a period of 7 months. This length of care for a wild animal may have too costly with conventional veterinary medicine and the animal may have been euthanized. Instead it was cured with affordable ethnoveterinary remedies and released.

The measurements are presented in metric where possible. It was not possible to accurately convert the herbal measurements such as teaspoons into grams without reweighing the actual herbs used at the time, so the quantities are represented in mls. The validation process also incorporates clinical studies and other clinical trials conducted on humans. This fits into the concept of "one medicine". This concept was first outlined by Sir William Osler one of the founders of medical teaching. It was later championed by veterinary epidemiologist Calvin Schwabe, DVM, MPH, ScD who was also a pioneer in ethnoveterinary medicine. Dr. Schwabe did not succeed in making the concept widespread but the campaign has now been embraced by Roger Mahr DVM the AVMA president and Ronald Davis the AMA President.

Methodology

The ethnoveterinary data collection took place over a six-month period. The sample size chosen was sixty. Two visits were made to each participant. Reliable information came from participants with years of experience. A draft outline of the participant's ethnoveterinary remedies was delivered and discussed at the second research visit in order to establish that dosages were accurately noted, for input on content, and to clarify any points. The participant-approved drafts were compiled into a draft manual and discussed at the workshop. Telephone interviews were conducted with participants whose location was distant from the research area to collect the relevant information. The draft outline was then posted to the relevant location and a second phone interview confirmed the data collected in the first. Medicinal plant specimens were collected where possible and were identified and deposited as vouchers in the University of Victoria herbarium.

Validation of practices

The research assistant and the ethnoveterinary consultant completed the non-experimental validation of the remedies in advance of the workshop. Only large drug companies can afford traditional validation. This research evaluated the ethnoveterinary plants used with a non-experimental method. This method consists of:

1. obtaining an accurate botanical identification

2. determining whether the folk data can be understood in terms of bioscientific concepts and methods

3. searching the pharmaceutical/ pharmacological literature for the plant's known chemical constituents and to determine the known physiological effects of either the crude plant, related species, or isolated chemical compounds that the plant is known to contain. This information is used to assess whether the plant use is based on empirically verifiable principles. For example if the plant is reputed to cause itching or bleeding, the assessment determines if it contains chemicals that can cause itching and bleeding.

If ethnobotanical data and pharmacological information supports the folk use of a plant species like *Aloe vera* above, it can be grouped into the validation level with the highest degree of confidence. Four levels of validity were used:

1. If no information supports the use it indicates that the plant may be inactive.

2. A plant (or closely related species of the same genus), which is used in geographically or temporally distinct areas in the treatment of similar illnesses, attains the lowest level of

validity, if no further phytochemical or pharmacological information validates the popular use. Use in other areas increases the likelihood that the plant is active against the illness.

3. If in addition to the ethnobotanical data, phytochemical or pharmacological information also validates the use in British Columbia, the plant may exert a physiological action on the patient and is more likely to be effective than those at the lowest level of validity.

4. If ethnobotanical and pharmacological data supports the folk use of the plant, it is grouped in the highest level of validity and is most likely an effective remedy.

VALIDATION WORKSHOP

The workshop involved participatory documentation and validation of the previously recorded ethnoveterinary remedies. Workshops offer an opportunity for the non-experimental validation of ethnoveterinary practices because scientists are able to discuss details of a local practice with the farmers familiar with them, compare these practices to standard veterinary methods and judge their applicability and effectiveness. Respondent participation is said to ensure better communication between scientists and respondents and increases the utility and reliability of the information that is reaching respondents.

Ten participants with experience in traditional human and ethnoveterinary medicine took part in the participatory five-day-long workshop at the University of Victoria (BC) in October, 2003. In the workshop the facilitator asked participants very specific questions in a supportive environment about the medicinal plants used. Some people did need others to be encouraged to talk and to refresh their memories about plants, uses and dosages. The group interview recognized that attitudes and perceptions are often developed through interaction with other people and individuals may shift due to the influence of others comments. Alternatively, some opinions may be held with certainty.

Each animal/livestock species was covered in a morning or afternoon session. At each session the participants (a different group each day to facilitate respondents' busy schedules) introduced themselves and their work and were acquainted with the participatory workshop method. The participants discussed the previously produced topic-specific parts of the manual. The practices chosen for inclusion in the manual were those that workshop participants and researchers considered to be safe and effective. There were editorial assistants/facilitators in attendance. After the first presentations and discussions, the materials were edited. This draft was then critiqued and modified by the group. This process was repeated on each day of the workshop.

For the pet session, one ethnobotanist, one holistic veterinarian and two herbalists were present. There were two editorial assistants/facilitators in attendance. After the discussions, the pet section of the results was edited. Two pet herbalists in the Vancouver Island community of Port Alberni were visited by the consultant and the first author and the edited pet data was discussed with them.

MANUAL OF TRADITIONAL PRACTICES

The final manual consisted of 180 pages covering diseases and treatments for horses (pgs 1 – 27), pets (28 – 81), pigs (84), poultry (85 – 94), rabbits (96 – 98) and ruminants (100 – 146). It was printed by Fotoprint, Pandora St, Victoria, BC.

A glossary and the introductory section called Part 1 (covering how to treat animals) were adapted with permission from *A Field Manual of Camel Diseases*, ITDG Publishing 103-105 Southampton Row London WC1B 4HL United Kingdom.

Editing was done by research assistant Cheryl Lans, ethnoveterinary consultant Dr Evelyn Mathias, research participant/farmer Jan Bevan and veterinarian Dr Tonya Khan.

Drawings were contributed by research participant Willi Boepple and UVic research associate Dr Fang Zhang.

The workshop was facilitated by Dr Rachel Westfall, UVic postdoctoral scholar in Sociology, and Bryce Gilroy-Scott, a UVic alumnus.

The manual was sent to all the participants, two copies went to the UVic library and one copy to a faculty veterinarian at the University of Guelph. Copies were also sent to Adam Davies ITDG publishing, Ilse Köhler-Rollefson the editor of *The Field Manual of Camel Diseases* and to Dr. Susan Wynn a leading consultant-ethnoveterinarian based in the US.

Acknowledgements

Professor Nancy Turner. Ethnobotanist at the University of Victoria, British Columbia, provided preliminary editing of the chapters in this book.

References

AVMNews: Editorial – Aug 13, 2007. Veterinarians and physicians: Working together for one medicine. Online at http://www.ama-assn.org/amednews/2007/08/13/edsa0813.htm

Bevan J, Lans C, Mathias M. (Eds). 2004. Alternative animal health care in British Columbia. A manual of traditional practices used by herbalists, veterinarians, farmers and animal caretakers. The Traditional Animal Health Care Collaborative. University of Victoria.

CBC News, 2002. Health Canada to examine livestock drugs Last Updated Thu, 25 Apr 2002 22:36:14. Internet address: http://cbc.ca/stories/2002/04/...

CBC Ottawa, 2002. Superbugs pose super cost Oct 8 2002 07:50 AM CDTottawa.cbc.ca/template/servlet/View?filename=superbugs021008 - 2002-10-08

Hadani, A., Shimshong, A. 1994. Traditional veterinary medicine in the Near East: Jews, Arab Bedouins and Fellahs. Rev. Sci. Tech. 13, 581 - 597.

Lans C, Turner N, Khan T. 2008. Medicinal plant treatments for fleas and ear problems of cats and dogs in British Columbia, Canada. Parasitology Research 103 (4): 889-898.

Lans C, Turner N, Khan T, Brauer G.2007. Ethnoveterinary medicines used to treat endoparasites and stomach problems in pigs and pets in British Columbia, Canada. Veterinary Parasitology 148: 325–340.

Lans C, Turner N, Khan T, Brauer G, Boepple W. 2007. Ethnoveterinary medicines used for ruminants in British Columbia, Canada. Journal of Ethnobiology and Ethnomedicine 3(1):11.

Lans C, Turner N, Brauer G, Lourenco G, and Georges K. 2006. Ethnoveterinary medicines used for horses in Trinidad and in British Columbia, Canada. Journal of Ethnobiology and Ethnomedicine 2 (1): 31.

Ethnoveterinary medicine (EVM) is the scientific term for traditional animal health care, and provides low-cost alternatives to allopathic drugs (Lans et al., 2006). All over the world, people who keep livestock have developed their own ideas and techniques of treating and managing their animals in a sustainable way. Many non-Western traditions of veterinary medicine exist, such as acupuncture and herbal medicine in China, Tibetan veterinary medicine, Ayurveda in India, etc. These traditions have written records that go back thousands of years, for example the Jewish sources in the Old Testament and Talamud and the Sri Lankans 400-year-old palm-leaf frond records of veterinary treatments (Hadani and Shimshony, 1994). Since colonial times scientists had always taken note of indigenous knowledge of animal health and diagnostic skills before implementing their Western-technology projects. EVM differs from this paternal approach by considering the traditional practices legitimate and seeking to validate them (Köhler-Rollefson and Bräunig, 1998).

EVM in future may be increasingly linked to discussions and research on ecosystem health. Ecosystem health is the study of the interconnections and relationships between livestock, environment and human health. Livestock management can enhance (brush control) or degrade the environment in various ways (overgrazing, water contamination). Medicinal plants are often collected in the wild and their continued supply depends on the continued existence of rainforests, secondary forests and other wild places (Giday, 2003).

EVM already has links to biodiversity conservation, for example Heifer Project International is establishing gardens of veterinary medical plants in Cameroon. Nomads in Iran collect the seeds of preferred forage species and put them in linen bags hung around the necks of the sheep leading the flock. During grazing, the seeds drop from the holes in the bottom of the bags and are worked into the ground by the hooves of the rest of the flock (Mathias, 2004).

EVM is now increasingly integrated into 'participatory epidemiology' which seeks to improve epidemiological surveillance in remote areas and encourage community participation in disease control (Mathias, 2004). EVM is also studied to provide solutions to diseases in which antigen variation has made vaccination unrealistic and drug resistant strains to Western medicines have become prevalent (Atawodi, 2002).

In 2003 participatory research was started on the ethnoveterinary remedies used in British Columbia, Canada (BC) (Lans et al., 2007). The research documented and validated (in a non-experimental way) the medicinal plants used by pet owners, holistic veterinarians and farmers. These chapters focus on the plants used for health problems in dogs, cats and one raccoon.

1. Materials and methods

1.1. Data collection

Ethnoveterinary data for British Columbia was collected for food (cows, goats, sheep, pigs) and companion animals (dogs, cats, horses and one raccoon) over a six-month period in 2003 and analyzed in the subsequent months. All available literature about livestock farmers and the secondary literature on ethnomedicinal plants, folk medicine and related fields in British Columbia was reviewed prior to and during the research. The research area included south Vancouver Island, the Lower Mainland, and the Thompson/Okanagan region of the Interior, the most populated regions (Lans et al., 2007).

A purposive sample of livestock farmers and pet owners was established to obtain the key informants holding the ethnoveterinary knowledge. The sample size chosen was 60 and this size was dictated by financial considerations. The sample was obtained from membership lists of organic farmers, other specialists in alternative medicine and holistic veterinarians. The majority of the information on pets came from two naturopaths, ten herbalists, five dog trainers, breeders and pet shop owners, nine holistic veterinarians and the majority of 27 organic farmers who had pets.

Two visits were made by Cheryl Lans with either Crystal Ross or Joanne Breckenridge to each farm, veterinary clinic or respondent. All of the initial interviews were open-ended and unstructured. A draft outline of the respondents' ethnoveterinary remedies from these interviews was then prepared, delivered and subsequently discussed during a second visit in order to confirm the data provided at the initial interview and to obtain more details on the treatments. Telephone interviews were conducted with participants whose location was too distant to collect the relevant information in person. The draft outline was then posted to the relevant respondent and a second phone interview confirmed the data collected in the first phone interview. Medicinal plant voucher specimens were collected whenever possible and were identified and deposited in the University of Victoria Herbarium (UVIC).

The plant-based remedies were evaluated for safety and efficacy with a non-experimental method, prior to including them in the draft outline and in the final manual. This evaluation process then continued throughout the data collection until the publication of the results. Journal articles, books and databases on pharmacology, ethnoveterinary medicine and ethnomedicine available on the Internet (PubMed, Science Direct) were searched to identify the plants' chemical compounds and clinically tested physiological effects. This data was incorporated with data on similar folk practices from, Asia, North America and Europe (Lans et al., 2007).

2.1.Non-experimental validation of ethnoveterinary remedies

Herbal remedies used for hundreds of years by stockraisers can be put to commercial use, but scientists within and outside the discipline are increasing demanding that traditional knowledge should be validated, to verify the safety and efficacy of the treatments. Also, the purpose of validation must be considered. For example will the end product serve the needs of the local population? Dr. Cheryl Lans and the ethnoveterinary consultant, Dr. Evelyn Mathias completed the majority of the non-experimental validation of the remedies in advance of the workshop. This method consisted of:

• obtaining an accurate botanical identification of the medicinal plants that were collected; and

• searching the pharmaceutical/pharmacological literature for the plant's identified chemical constituents in order to determine the known physiological effects of either the crude plant drug, related species, or isolated chemical compounds that the plant is known to contain. This information was then used to assess whether the plant use might be based on empirically verifiable principles.

Supporting ethnobotanical data and pharmacological information was matched with the recorded folk use of the plant species, to determine degrees of confidence about its effectiveness. Four levels of confidence were used:

1. Minimal: no information supports the use, indicating that the plant may be inactive; a plant (or closely related species of the same genus), which is used in geographically or temporally distinct areas in the treatment of similar illnesses, attains the minimal level of validity, if no further phytochemical or pharmacological information validates the popular use. Use in other areas increases the likelihood that the plant is active against the illness.

2. A plant (or closely related species of the same genus), which is used in geographically or temporally distinct areas in the treatment of similar illnesses, attains the lowest level of validity, if no further phytochemical or pharmacological information validates the popular use. Use in other areas increases the likelihood that the plant is active against the illness.

3. If, in addition to the ethnobotanical data, phytochemical or pharmacological information is also known from a species in British Columbia, this is further indication that the plant may exert a physiological action on the patient and is considered more likely to be effective than those at the lowest level of validity.

4. High level: If ethnobotanical, phytochemical or pharmacological and clinical trial data are consistent with the ethnoveterinary use of the plant; its use is classed in the highest level of validity and it is considered highly probably to be efficacious.

TABLE 1. NON-EXPERIMENTAL VALIDATION FOR ALOE VERA

Scientific name	Published literature	Chemical constituents
Aloe vera	Karaca *et al.*, 1995. Chinnah *et al.*, 1992; Davis *et al.*, 1994; Lal jawahar *et al.*, 1990; Afzal *et al.*, 1991	Acemannan, a polydispersed $\beta(1\text{-}4)$-linked acetylated mannan, enhances the immune response to both Newcastle Disease Virus and Infectious Bursal Disease Virus.

2.2 Validation workshop

Ten participants with experience in folk and ethnoveterinary medicine took part in a five-day-long participatory workshop at the University of Victoria (BC) in October, 2003. During the workshop the facilitator asked the participants detailed questions in a supportive environment about the medicinal plants used, for example in order to clarify details on dosage and preparation. Each animal/livestock species was discussed in a morning or afternoon session -- other than the core group, different participants with different specialties came to different sessions. The pet data was evaluated by an ethnobotanist, a holistic veterinarian and two herbalists. There were two editorial assistants/facilitators in attendance at all sessions. After the discussions, the pet section of the results was edited and included into a manual that was given to all the research participants at the end of the study (TAHCC, 2004).

Results

Many of the treatments were given in imperial measurements during the interviews. These measurements were changed to approximate metric measurements but the original imperial measurements for the herbal materials are retained for accuracy. The results for ethnoveterinary remedies used for pets are published in the subsequent chapters of this volume. Results previously published can be obtained from the papers in the reference list.

Acknowledgements
The research in British Columbia was funded by the Social Sciences and Humanities Research Council of Canada (SSHRC) Grant # 820-2002-1008. Dr. Evelyn Mathias provided professional support. We are grateful to the Herbarium at the University of Victoria, and to all of the research participants. Research participants Jan Bevan and Sheelagh MacKenzie-Salas collected botanical voucher specimens and we appreciate this. UVic alumni Joanne Breckenridge and Crystal Ross also collected botanical voucher specimens.

References

Adger, W. Neil, 2000. Social and ecological resilience: Are they related? Progress in Human Geography 24 (3), 347 – 364.

Afzal, M., Ali. M., Hassan. R.A.H., Sweedan, N., Dhami, M.S.I. 1991. Identification of some prostanoids in *Aloe vera* extracts. Planta Medica 57, 38-40.

Atawodi, S.E., Ameh, D.A., Ibrahim, S., Andrew, J.N., Nzelibe, H.C., Onyike, E.O., Anigo, K.M., Abu, E.A., James, D.B., Njoku, G.C., Sallau, A.B. 2002. Indigenous knowledge system for treatment of trypanosomiasis in Kaduna state of Nigeria. J Ethnopharmacol 79 (2): 279-82.

Browner, C.H., Ortiz de Montellano, B.R., Rubel, A.J., 1988. A methodology for cross-cultural ethnomedical research. Current Anthropology 29, 681 – 702.

Browner, C.H., Ortiz de Montellano, B.R., Rubel, A.J., 1988. A methodology for cross-cultural ethnomedical research. Current Anthropology 29, 681 – 702.

CBC News, 2002. Health Canada to examine livestock drugs Last Updated Thu, 25 Apr 2002 22:36:14. Internet address: http://cbc.ca/stories/2002/04/...

CBC Ottawa, 2002. Superbugs pose super cost Oct 8 2002 07:50 AM CDTottawa.cbc.ca/template/servlet/View?filename=superbugs021008 - 2002-10-08

Chinnah, A.D., Baig, M.A., Tizard, I.R., Kemp, M.C. 1992. Antigen dependent adjuvant activity of a polydispersed β-(1-4)-linked acetylated mannan (acemannan). Vaccine 10 (8), 551 - 557.

Croom, E.M. Jr. 1983. Documenting and evaluating herbal remedies. Economic Botany 37 (1), 13 - 27.

Dakers, Sonya. 1992. Sustainable agriculture: Future dimensions. Ottawa: Library of Parliament, Research Branch.

Davis, R.H., Donato, J.J., Hartman, G.M., Haas, R.C. 1994. Anti-inflammatory and wound healing activity of a growth substance in *Aloe vera*. Journal of the American Podiatric Medical Assoc. 84 (2), 77 - 81.

Duram, Leslie, A., Larson, Kelli, L. 2001. Agricultural research and alternative farmers' information needs. Professional Geographer 53 (1), 84 – 96.

Giday, M., Asfaw, Z., Elmqvist, T., Woldu, Z. 2003. An ethnobotanical study of medicinal plants used by the Zay people in Ethiopia. J Ethnopharmacol 85: 43 - 52.

Heinrich, M., Rimpler, H., Antonio-Barrerra, N., 1992. Indigenous phytotherapy of gastrointestinal disorders in a lowland Mixe community (Oaxaca, Mexico): Ethnopharmacologic evaluation. Journal of Ethnopharmacology 36, 63 - 80.

Hirschhorn, H. 1983. Constructing a phytotherapeutic concordance based upon Tropical American and Indonesian examples. Journal of Ethnopharmacology 7 (2), 157 - 167.

IIRR, 1994. Ethnoveterinary medicine in Asia: An information kit on traditional animal health care practices. 4 Vols. International Institute of Rural Reconstruction, Silang, Cavite, Philippines.

IIRR, 1996. Recording and using indigenous knowledge: A manual. International Institute of Rural Reconstruction, Silang, Cavite, Philippines.

ITDG and IIRR, 1996. Ethnoveterinary medicine in Kenya: A field manual of traditional animal health care practices. Nairobi, Kenya: Intermediate Technology Development Group and International Institute of Rural Reconstruction.

Karaca, K., Sharma, J.M., Nordgren, R. 1995. Nitric oxide production by chicken macrophages activated by acemannan, a complex carbohydrate extracted from *Aloe vera*. Int. J. Immunopharmac. 17 (3), 183 -188.

Köhler-Rollefson, Ilse and Bräunig, Juliane, 1998. Anthropological Veterinary Medicine: The Need for Indigenizing the Curriculum. Paper presented at the 9th AITVM Conference in Harare, 14th-18th September, 1998.

Lans, C., Turner, N., Brauer, G., Lourenco, G., Georges, K. 2006. Ethnoveterinary medicines used for horses in Trinidad and in British Columbia, Canada. Journal of Ethnobology and Ethnomedicine 2:31.

Lans, C., Turner, N., Khan, T., Brauer, G., 2007. Ethnoveterinary medicines used to treat endoparasites and stomach problems in pigs and pets in British Columbia, Canada. Vet. Parasitol 148, 325–340.

Mackinnon, Andy, and Jim Pojar (Eds.). 1994. Plants of Coastal British Columbia including Washington, Oregon and Alaska. Lone Pine Publishing, Vancouver and Edmonton. (Ethnobotanical contributions by N. Turner and A. Reed).

MacRae, R.J., Hill, S.B., Henning, J. and Bentley, A.J. 1990. Policies, programs and regulations to support the transition to sustainable agriculture in Canada. American Journal of Alternative Agriculture 5 (2), 76-92.

Mathias-Mundy, E. 1996. How can ethnoveterinary medicine be used in field projects? Indigenous Knowledge and Development Monitor 4 (2), 6 - 7.

Mathias-Mundy, Evelyn and McCorkle, C.M. 1989. Ethnoveterinary Medicine: An Annotated Bibliography. Bibliographies in Technology and Social Change No. 6. Iowa State U, Ames, Iowa, USA.

Mathias, E. 2004. Ethnoveterinary medicine: Harnessing its potential. Vet Bull 74 (8): 27N – 37N.

Mundy, Paul and Evelyn Mathias. 1997. Participatory workshops to produce information materials on ethnoveterinary medicine. Paper presented at the International Conference on Ethnoveterinary Medicine: Alternatives for Livestock Development, Pune, India, 4–6 November 1997.

Raedeke, Andrew, H., Rikoon, Sanford, J. 1997. Temporal and spatial dimensions of knowledge: Implications for sustainable agriculture. Agriculture and Human Values 14, 145 – 158.

Select Standing Committee on Agriculture and Fisheries. 1999. Transcript of Proceedings, Issue No. 20. 1998/99 Legislative Session: 3rd Session, 36th Parliament (October 12). Victoria, BC: Queen's Printer. Available Internet: http://www.legis.gov.bc.ca/cmt/36thparl/cmt08/hansard/1999/af101299.htm

TAHCC, 2004. Alternative Animal Health Care in British Columbia: A manual of traditional practices used by herbalists, veterinarian, farmers and animal caretakers. The Traditional Animal Health Care Collaborative. Victoria, British Columbia, Canada.

Turner, Nancy J. (ed.). 1992. Plants for All Reasons: Culturally Important Plants of Aboriginal Peoples of Southern Vancouver Island. Environmental Studies Program, University of Victoria, Teaching Manual, written by students of Environmental Studies 400C Class and University Extension Class, July 1992.

Turner, Nancy J. and Brian D. Compton. 1991. A Short Guide to Interviewing and Collecting Plants for Ethnobotanical Purposes. Report to Secwepemc Cultural Education Society, Simon Fraser Program, Environmental Studies 416, UVic.

Turner, Nancy J., Laurence C. Thompson, M. Terry Thompson and Annie Z. York. 1990. Thompson Ethnobotany. Knowledge and Usage of Plants by the Thompson Indians of British Columbia. Royal British Columbia Museum, Memoir No. 3, Victoria, British Columbia (335 pp.). Turner, Nancy J. 1995. Food Plants of Coastal First Peoples. Royal British Columbia

Museum Handbook, Victoria, B.C. (revised from 1975 edition, Food Plants of British Columbia

Indians. Part 1. Coastal Peoples), University of British Columbia Press, 164 pp.

Van Kessel, Henry, 2001. B.C. farming at a disadvantage. Agri Digest 17 (4).

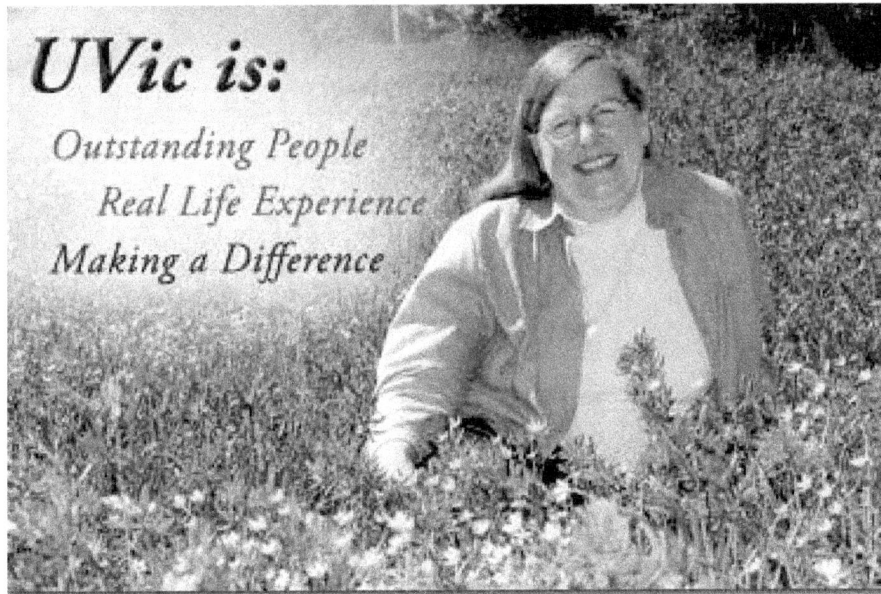

UVic's Dr. Nancy Turner http://communications.uvic.ca

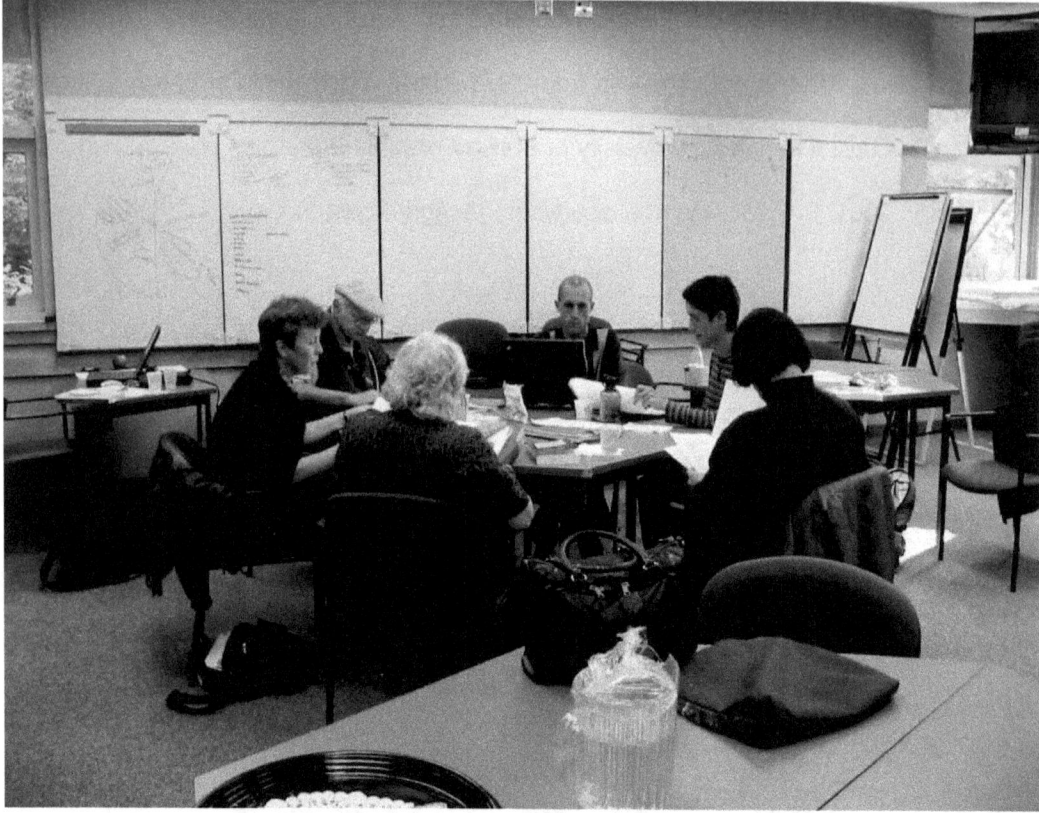

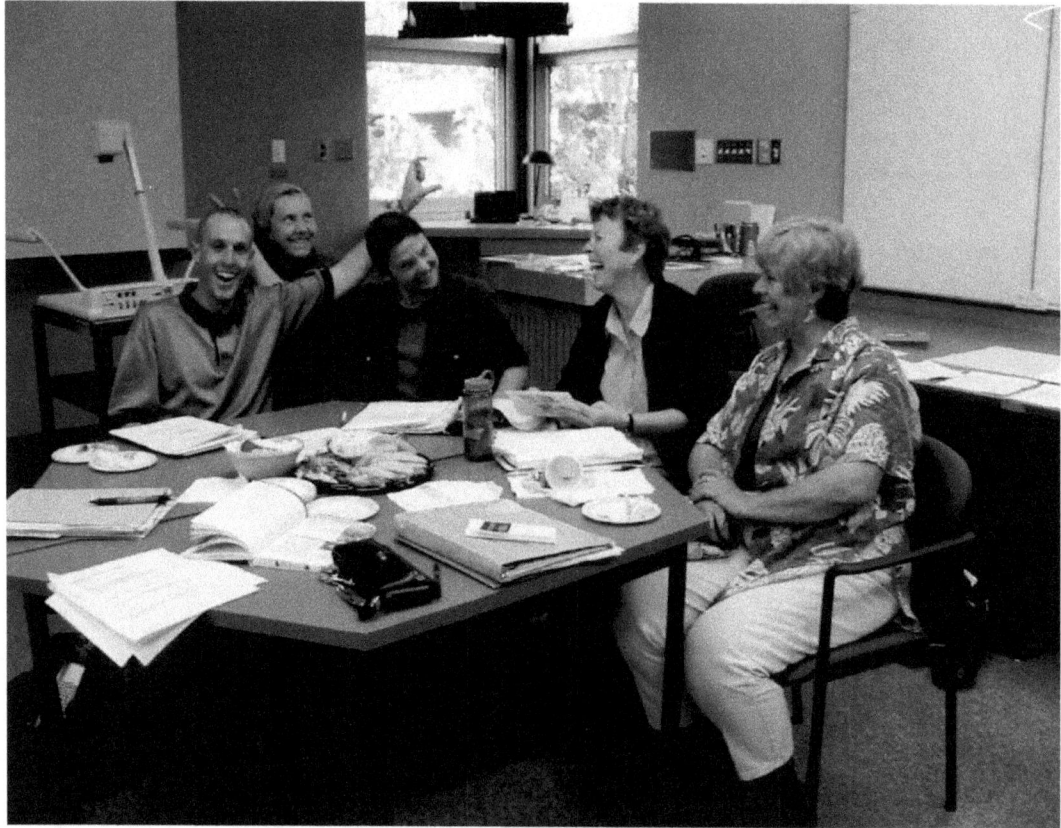

Abstract

This chapter deals with the medicinal plants used to treat injuries and arthritis in pets in British Columbia, Canada. The injuries treated include abscesses, sprains and abrasions. Treatment of dogs with rheumatoid arthritis, joint pain and articular cartilage injuries with plant-based remedies are also reported.

Anal gland problems are treated with *Allium sativum* L. (Liliaceae), *Aloe vera* L. (Liliaceae), *Calendula officinalis* L. (Asteraceae), *Plantago major* L. (Plantaginaceae), *Ulmus fulva* Michx. (Ulmaceae), *Urtica dioica* L. (Urticaceae) and the lichen *Usnea longissima* Ach. (Parmeliaceae). Antioxidants in plants, such as diarctigenin from *Arctium lappa*, used in our research for rheumatoid arthritis and joint pain in pet are said to be of use in treating pathological conditions such as inflammation and rheumatoid arthritis that are linked to excess production of reactive oxygen species.

Keywords: arthritis; injuries; pets; British Columbia; medicinal plants; ethnoveterinary medicine

1. Introduction

Ethnoveterinary medicine (EVM) is the scientific term for traditional animal health care, and provides low-cost alternatives to allopathic drugs (Lans et al., 2006). This chapter reports on the ethnoveterinary remedies used by small-scale, organic livestock farmers, holistic veterinarians and pet owners in British Columbia (B.C.), Canada.

This chapter deals specifically with the medicinal plants used to treat pets with injuries such as abscesses, bleeding wounds, sprains, post-operative bleeding, deep wounds, abrasions, arthritis, rheumatoid arthritis, joint pain and articular cartilage injuries.

Respondents provided several remedies for companion animal injuries. Cats often have abscesses or infected wounds obtained during fights; these are cleaned by veterinarians and a narrow spectrum antimicrobial agent is prescribed (Roy et al., 2007). The most common bacteria found in these wounds are *Pasteurella multocida* , *Streptococcus canis*, *Staphylococcus intermedius*, *Corynebacterium* spp., *Enterococcus* spp., and obligate anaerobes – *Prevotella melaninogenica/oralis, Prevotella bivida, Prevotella intermedia, Fusobacterium necrophorum/ nucleatum, Fusobacteriium varium, Fusobacterium* spp., *Porphyromonas asaccharolytica, Bacteroides uniformis, Bacteroides stercoris, Bacteroides vulgatus, Bacteroides fragilis* and *Bacteroides* sp.

Osteoarthritis is a painful musculoskeletal disorder distinguished by structural and functional changes in joint tissues, including articular cartilage loss, inflammation of the synovium lining of the joints and bone sclerosis (Rossetti et al., 1997; Henrotin, 2005; Henrotin et al., 2006). The loss of articular cartilage is due to an imbalance between synthesis and degradation of the extracellular cartilage matrix (Schulze-Tanzil et al., 2004). Arthritis and osteoarthritis diseases are accompanied by an increased induction of cytokines such as interleukin 1beta (IL-1beta) and tumor necrosis factor alpha (TNF-alpha). This in turn leads to an enhanced production of matrix-degrading enzymes (the matrix metalloproteinases (MMPs).

Secondary osteoarthritis can develop from joint dysplasia, osteochondrosis dissecans (damaged or abnormal cartilage), ununited anconeal process (elbow dysplasia) and patellar luxation (knee cap displacement). Acquired musculoskeletal disorders can lead to progressive cartilage deterioration. The initial lesion that develops from a trauma incident can become an extended and progressive degenerative lesion.

After ligamentous injuries, cartilage lesions may form due to joint instability. Joint luxation or luxation reduction are commonly associated with ligament and capsule damage and/or cartilage lesions. Mechanical injuries can lead to osteochondral microfractures, abnormal bone and cartilage remodelling with the final stage being cartilage loss and bone sclerosis. The synovial tissue is also activated. Excessive release of matrix components or broken particles from the damaged cartilage can activate synovial macrophages and fibroblasts, which then generates an extensive array of catabolic factors that lead to further degradation (Henrotin, 2005; Henrotin et al., 2006).

Osteoarthritic chondrocytes show an altered phenotype characterized by an excess production of catabolic factors, including metalloproteinases (i.e. collagenases, aggrecanases and stromelysin-1) and reactive oxygen species (hydrogen peroxide, superoxide anions, nitric oxide, peroxynitrite) (Henrotin, 2005; Henrotin et al., 2006).

Rheumatic disorders can originate from inflammatory, metabolic, degenerative or infectious causes (Grube et al., 2007). Rheumathoid arthritis is typified by synovial inflammation in the joints. A complex response of chemical mediators, chemotactic factors, leukocytes and phagocytes cause injury to cartilage and other tissues (Rotelli et al., 2003). The proliferation of the synovial lining layer causes environmental changes that result in low oxygen conditions (hypoxia) (Westra et al., 2007). The immunopathogenesis of rheumathoid arthritis can be eased with omega-3 fatty acids (gammalinolenic acid) (from fish oil and olive oil) (Rossetti et al., 1997; Khanna et al., 2007). Numerous plant-compounds can suppress the cell signaling intermediates involved in arthritis, including quercetin and rosmarinic acid (Rotelli et al., 2003; Khanna et al., 2007; Hur et al., 2007; Youn et al., 2003). Rutin was shown to be effective in experimental animal models of arthritis (Rotelli et al., 2003). Studies have shown good evidence of antiinflammatory activity for many of the ethnoveterinary plants used in this chapter such as devil's claw (*Harpagophytum procumbens*), white willow (*Salix alba*), comfrey (*Symphytum officinale*) , nettles (*Urtica dioica*), skullcap (*Scutellaria lateriflora*), and burdock (*Arctium lappa*) (Pearson et al., 2007).

2. Materials and methods

The methods used to document these remedies are described in the introductory chapter.

3. Results

Table 2 contains the ethnoveterinary plants used for various injuries and anal gland problems in pets in British Columbia. Table 3 includes the medicinal plants used for rheumatoid arthritis, joint pain and articular cartilage injuries.

Treatment for dog bites

Pets are given purchased tinctures orally of the following herbs for at least five days after a dog bite: Echinacea (*Echinacea purpurea*), goldenseal (*Hydrastis canadensis*), comfrey (*Symphytum officinalis*), calendula (*Calendula officinalis*) and astragalus (*Astragalus membranaceous*) (1 drop per 0.45 kg body weight of each herb). A tincture or an olive oil infusion of St. John's Wort

(*Hypericum perforatum*) flowers is used orally and externally (1 to 2 drops per 6.8 kg bodyweight) as the only treatment with no other herbs being utilised. In the manual we cautioned that puncture wounds in cats should be monitored to make sure that they stayed open; healing from the inside out. Puncture wounds are flushed with warm saline solution, then bathed the wound with saline solution plus ½-1 drop tincture of calendula (*Calendula officinalis*) for the duration of the healing process. Pets are also given 1 drop of calendula tincture (*Calendula officinalis*) per 5 kg bodyweight, orally.

Treatment of dental problems

One dog was recommended for oral surgery because of a gum inflammation due to a broken tooth. Instead a tincture of myrrh (*Commiphora molmol*) diluted to 50% was dropped on the gum twice a day for four days to alleviate the gum infection. The same diluted tincture (30 to 40 drops in water) was also used by respondents as a rinse for deep abscesses and was supplemented with the following– 60 ml (¼ cup) sage (*Salvia officinalis*), 60 ml (¼ cup) calendula flower, 60 ml (¼ cup) rose hips (*Rosa* sp.).

Treatment for a raccoon in a coma

An adult female raccoon, 6.8 kg, not neutered, was involved in a car accident resulting in central nervous system damage. She was in a coma with unknown injuries to the brain, blindness, her muscles were completely rigid and her hands were locked in a clenched position. She had no movement. The raccoon was given species-appropriate food and hydrotherapy treatments in order to increase her mobility. She was considered well after seven months. These tinctures were given to the raccoon:

Concentration	Tincture 1	Tincture 2	Tincture 3

Total mls		100 ml	25 ml	120 ml
Avena sativa seeds and whole plant	1:5/25%	20 ml	10 ml	25 ml
Hypericum perforatum aerial flowering parts	1:5/45%; 2:5/25% (tinctures 2&3)	20 ml	10 ml	25 ml
Scutellaria lateriflora aerial parts	2:5/25%	10 ml	n/a	15 ml
Ginkgo biloba leaves	1:5/25%	5 ml	n/a	5 ml
Eleutherococcus senticosus dried root	1:5/25%	5 ml	n/a	25 ml
Medicago sativa	1:4/ 25%	20 ml	n/a	n/a
Vegetable glycerine		20 ml	n/a	20 ml
Centella asiatica aerial parts	1:5/ 25%	5 ml	n/a	n/a
Fagus sylvatica flower essence		2 drops	2 drops	2 drops
Rescue remedy		n/a	2 drops	2 drops
			Started 2 months after tincture 1 with 10 ml left in the bottle	
Administration		15 drops mixed into the food twice a day for 66 days	15 drops mixed into the food twice a day for 23 days	15 drops mixed into the food twice a day for 80 days

Treatment for bleeding wounds, sprains, post-operative bleeding, deep wounds, abrasions

Injuries are treated with a rinse or soak of Epsom salts mixed with water. Subsequently a commercial calendula gel or flush (*Calendula officinalis*) is used for external treatment. If a wound is clean, and not likely to be infected the following plants are used in 1.36 litres of water to make a wash or salve: 80 ml (1/3 cup) cut plantain leaf, 80 ml (1/3 cup) cut comfrey leaf and 80 ml (1/3 cup) packed calendula flowers.

Infected wounds were washed twice daily with an antimicrobial-substitute tea made with any or all of the following: Oregon grape (*Berberis aquifolium*/*Mahonia aquifolium*), St John's wort (*Hypericum perforatum*), 5 ml (½ tsp) dried leaves goldenseal (*Hydrastis canadensis*), and 5 ml (½ tsp) myrrh (*Commiphora molmol*). When the infection was resolved, a comfrey/plantain/calendula salve was used on the wound.

A solution of 1 part tea tree oil (*Melaleuca alternifolia*) mixed with 9 parts olive oil was applied to a cotton ball and dabbed straight onto wounds, bites, rashes, vaccination sites and stings to help healing and discomfort. Calendula ointment (*Calendula officinalis*) was used on closed wounds. Calendula tea or diluted tincture was used on open wounds (10 to 12 drops of tincture in 0.23 litres of water per 22.7 to 27.2 kg bodyweight). An infusion with oil of St. John's Wort (*Hypericum perforatum*) was used on surgery scars. A poultice for wounds was made with 45 ml (3 tbsp) slippery elm bark powder (*Ulmus fulva*) with 0.23 litres of water. Self heal (*Prunella vulgaris*) flowering aerial parts were crushed and put on wounds. One tsp (5 ml) plantain leaf (*Plantago major*) or comfrey leaves (*Symphytum officinalis*) were chewed and used as a poultice if pets were injured while on walks. A wound wash of myrrh gum resin (*Commiphora molmol, C. abyssinica, C. myrrha*) (2 ml or ½ tsp) was prepared by infusing the resin for ½ hour in 0.23 litres of water and this wash was dripped onto wounds. Echinacea roots (*Echinacea angustifolia, Echinacea purpurea, Echinacea pallida*) or a tea of 80 ml (1/3 cup) leaves in 0.46 litres of water were also used for wounds (18 – 20 kg bodyweight). Echinacea root tincture was given orally: 1 or 2 drops.

A lavender wound wash was made with 0.45 litres of distilled water, 2 oz vodka and 15 drops essential oil of lavender (*Lavandula officinalis*). One tbsp (15 ml) of this was used. Or a lavender infusion was used (5 – 10 ml or 1-2 tsp of dried lavender flowers in 0.23 litres of boiling water). Raspberry leaf tea (*Rubus idaeus, R. strigosus*) was also used to wash wounds (0.23 litres of boiling water on 5 ml (1 tsp) dried leaves). Raspberry leaves were also combined with 5 ml (1 tsp) slippery elm bark powder (*Ulmus fulva*) to wash wounds, or they were combined with myrrh. Another wound wash was made using the following: 30 ml (1/8 cup) of dried Echinacea root (*Echinacea purpurea* or *Echinacea pallida*), 15 ml (1 tbsp) dried self heal (*Prunella vulgaris*), 30 ml (1/8 cup) of dried oregano (*Origanum vulgaris*), 15 ml (1 tbsp) dried lavender flowers (*Lavandula angustifolia*), and 15 ml (1 tbs) dried calendula flowers (*Calendula officinalis*) (all chopped and used to fill 2/3 of a glass jar with vodka added to fill). A salve was made by adding the following to olive oil and beeswax: 15 ml (1 tbsp) fresh comfrey (*Symphytum officinalis*), 15 ml (1 tbsp) calendula (*Calendula officinalis*) flowers and 15 ml (1 tbsp) chickweed (*Stellaria media*). This salve was used to treat a dog whose nose was partially ripped off by a raccoon. The nose was reattached and healed without surgery.

Treatments for minor anal gland problem in dogs

Dogs with anal gland problems are given a changed diet (see below). A tea of nettles (*Urtica dioica*) was given as a drink or is mixed with food. Chopped garlic (*Allium sativum*) (1/3 clove) was added to the food. Slippery elm (*Ulmus fulva*) (10 ml or 2 tsp daily, in frequent doses) was added to moist food to aid in defecation. A nettles decoction (*Urtica dioica*) (2 oz of fresh chopped roots or 15 ml (1 tbsp) dried chopped roots in 0.57 litres of water) was given. Or nettles juice was made with an armful of nettles tops and administered.

Four drops of Rescue Remedy (Bach Flower) were given before treatment. Or 15 – 20 drops of calendula tincture (*Calendula officinalis*) were given every two to three hours for acute cases, 15 - 20 drops tincture (1 dropperful) of plantain (*Plantago major*) was also given orally. These tinctures were sometimes diluted before use. An optional addition to the treatment regimen consisted of 10 to 15 drops (1/2 dropperful) tincture of *Usnea* spp. External treatments consisted of one part tincture of calendula (*Calendula officinalis*) and 1 part tincture of plantain (*Plantago major*) which were applied to warm cotton already soaked in hot saline solution. Optionally one half-part tincture of *Usnea* spp., was used in addition to the above tinctures. These tinctures were applied with pressure directly to the wound for as long as the dog would allow and until the cloth was cool (5 min). While holding the cloth to the wound the dog was massaged on either side of its spine towards the tail. For acute conditions this treatment was given every two to three hours for three days, then three times a day until the sore healed. *Aloe vera* gel was added to the treatment in the final stages.

Emergency treatment for a snakebite

Pets are given an *Echinacea purpurea* tincture for snakebites (unspecified snake) (100 drops every 20 minutes until the tincture was finished). Or a poultice of chewed leaves of plantain (*Plantago major*) with echinacea tincture is used. Both plants are also administered as teas. Yellow dock (*Rumex crispus*) leaves are used when plantain was not available.

The following remedies are used for arthritis, bruising and rheumatoid arthritis

Pets are given Acadian sea kelp (*Fucus vesiculosus*) to provide trace minerals, fibre, chlorophyll and antioxidants. Small dogs are given 10 ml (2 tsp) of organic kelp/alfalfa (*Medicago sativa*) (1:1) mix per day as an antirheumatic and for joint pain. Medium to large breed dogs are given

30 ml (2 tbsp) kelp/alfalfa mix per day. Or 15 ml (1 tbsp) kelp per 45 kg of patient bodyweight every three days and 10 ml (2 tsp) dried alfalfa leaves every second day.

Other dogs are given 60 ml (1/4 cup) of a strained decoction per day as their drinking water per 11.3 kg patient bodyweight. The plants used were (5 ml or 1 heaping tsp each in 1.8 litres of water): devil's claw (*Harpagophytum procumbens*), nettle leaves (*Urtica dioica*), chaparral (*Larrea tridentata*), hydrangea root (*Hydrangea arborescens*), burdock root (*Arctium lappa*), wild lettuce (*Lactuca virosa*), lobelia (*Lobelia inflata*), sarsaparilla (*Smilax officinalis*), black cohosh (*Actaea/Cimicifuga racemosa*) and black walnut fruit hull (*Juglans nigra*). Added to these plants are Bentonite clay and cayenne pepper.

A horsetail tincture in apple cider vinegar is given every day (20 drops) for extended periods for its mineral content (silica). A 1:1 tincture or tea is used (5 drops daily for a month per 22.7 kg patient bodyweight). The treatments are then suspended for a month. The treatment is restarted for arthritis or to increase the mineral content of the diet, or for a broken bone. A cayenne tincture (purchased product) 1 to 5 drops, is also used for these conditions. This tincture is considered safe for pets to lick off. Alternatively a homemade paste is made with cayenne powder and vegetable oil and this is then rubbed on, after first testing it on the owner's wrist. The dose of glucosamine used for a 45.4 kg dog was 1 mg to 2 mg.

Treatment for a dog with an injury to the articular cartilage

The patient was a 34 kg dog that was eight months old. It was limping, had reduced motion, tenderness on touch, instability of the knee-joint and edema. The diet was adjusted to include supplements that support bone and muscle development. A salve of comfrey (*Symphytum officinalis* leaves and roots) was applied externally. This was used in combination with a tincture of comfrey (whole plant) applied directly on the injured area (1 to 5 drops twice a day) for five days. The treatment was suspended for two days then restarted. While the dog was on the comfrey treatment the meat protein in the diet was reduced. Rescue Remedy (Bach Flower Remedy) was given orally - 4 drops diluted in one glass of water, prior to administration of the salve medication or to keep the dog calm while the injury healed. Also given was a tincture of leaf and root of dandelion (*Taraxacum officinalis*) (15 drops three times a day until resolution). Additionally one gram (or fluid equivalent) of the bark of white willow (*Salix alba*) was given three times a day with food or with the tinctures for inflammation and pain.

Diet for a dog with articular cartilage injury

Nettles (*Urtica dioica*) 28 grams herb: with 0.51 litres of water was given as a tea. Or nettle capsules (210 mg) were given - 4 to 5 capsules once a day; alfalfa (*Medicago sativa*) – 250 mg once a day; garlic (*Allium sativum*) 1 fresh clove daily; white willow (*Salix alba*) – as above; kelp – 2 ml (1/2 tsp) for every 4.5 kg of body weight; sodium ascorbate – ongoing low dose during treatment, 250 – 500 mg, twice daily. If the stools are loose, the dose was reduced.

Treatment for a torn cruciate ligament

This treatment was used for partial tears of the cruciate ligament of a dog. An infusion was made with 30 ml (2 tbsp) snipped fresh leaves of comfrey (*Symphytum officinalis*) in 0.34 litres of boiling water 5 ml (1 tsp) strained liquid per 11.3 kg bodyweight for two weeks twice a day in the food). An infusion was made with 120 ml (½ cup) comfrey and 60 ml (¼ cup) alfalfa (*Medicago sativa*) in 0.45 litres of water. The infusion provided interim support until the date for surgery or it was used as a treatment for a minor torn cruciate ligament.

4. Discussion

The non-experimental validation of the plants is presented in Table 4. The validation process is explained in the introductory chapter.

Prunella vulgaris was used for wounds in dogs and cats in our study. An aqueous fraction of this plant inhibits anaphylactic shock, allergic reactions and protects rat erythrocytes against haemolysis and kidney and brain homogenates against lipid peroxidation (Psotová et al., 2003). Antimicrobial activity was also found. All of these findings support the ethnomedicinal use of *Prunella vulgaris* for ethnoveterinary wound healing and as an anti-inflammatory remedy. The wound healing effectiveness of Aloe (*Aloe barbadensis*) is well known. Calendula (*Calendula officinalis*) was given C grades for skin inflammation and wound healing by Basch et al., (2006) due to the paucity of studies. Lavender (*Lavandula angustifolia*), oregano (*Origanum vulgare*) and sage (*Salvia officinalis*) all contain ursolic acid (Duke, 2008). Ursolic acid can suppress tumourigenesis, inhibit tumour promotion and suppress angiogenesis (Shishodia et al., 2003). These effects are mediated through suppression of the expression of lipoxygenase, COX-2, MMP-9, and iNOS. Ursolic acid can suppress NF-KB activation induced by inflammatory agents and tumor promoters.

The dried root of *Astragalus membranaceus* enhances various types of immune responses such as phagocytic activity of macrophages, T cell activity and cytotoxicity of natural killer or lymphokine-activated killer cells (Shon and Nam, 2003). Astragaloside IV, a saponin purified from *Astragalus membranaceus* interferes with a major inflammatory pathway the NF-KB pathway (Zhang et al., 2003).

Chronic arthritis in humans or other animals can result from the dysregulation of pro-inflammatory cytokines (e.g. tumor necrosis factor and interleukin-1b) and pro-inflammatory enzymes that act on the production of prostaglandins (e.g. cyclooxygenase-2) and leukotrienes (e.g. lipooxygenase), along with the expression of adhesion molecules and matrix metalloproteinases, and the increased production of synovial fibroblasts. All of these factors are regulated by the activation of the transcription factor nuclear factor-kB. Therefore plant-based compounds that suppress the expression of tumour necrosis factor-a, interleukin-1b, cyclooxygenase-2, lipooxygenase, matrix metalloproteinases or adhesion molecules, or suppress the activation of NF-kB, are potential treatments for arthritis (Khanna et al., 2007). Table 5 lists the molecular targets of the ethnoveterinary remedies or constituent plant compounds that exhibit anti-arthritic potential.

Harpagophytum procumbens, *Salix alba*, and *Capsicum frutescens* were found to reduce pain (Gagnier et al., 2006; Gregory et al., 2008). An aqueous extract of *Harpagophytum procumbens* at a standardized daily dosage of 50 mg harpagoside had strong evidence for the short-term treatment of acute episodes of chronic nonspecific low back pain. An aqueous extract of *Harpagophytum procumbens* at a standardized daily dosage of 100 mg harpagoside (the active iridoid glycoside), had moderate evidence for the short-term treatment of acute episodes of chronic nonspecific low back pain: as did an extract of *Salix alba* at a standardized dosage of 120 mg salicin per day and two plasters of *Capsicum frutescens* (either a topical plaster application containing 11 mg of capsaicinoids per plaster, or a plaster containing an ethonolic extract of cayenne pepper standardized to 22 µg/cm^2 of capsaicinoinds).The antiinflammatory action of *Harpagophytum procumbens* is due to its action on eicosanoid biosynthesis (Settee and Sigal, 2005).

Black cohosh extracts (*Actaea racemosa*) have many biological activities including anticancer, anti-inflammatory, and antioxidant possibly due to the complex synergistic action of its components. A lignan, actaealactone, and a phenylpropanoid ester derivative, cimicifugic acid G, as well as 15 known polyphenols, were isolated from the rhizomes and roots of black cohosh (*Actaea racemosa*). Actaealactone and cimicifugic acid had antioxidant activity (Nuntanakorn et al., 2006).

5. Conclusion

The treatment of arthritis with nonsteroidal anti-inflammatory drugs (NSAIDs) does not block or reverse cartilage degradation and joint destruction and is associated with well known adverse effects therefore plant-based remedies may prove to be viable alternatives (Ahmed et al., 2005). Excess production of reactive oxygen species and other radicals have been suggested as inducers of tissue injury in many pathological conditions such as inflammation and rheumatoid arthritis (Choi and Hwang, 2005). Diarctigenin from *Arctium lappa*, used as an ethnoveterinary remedy for rheumatoid arthritis and joint pain in pets, strongly inhibited nitric oxide production (Park et al., 2007). In their experiment Pearson et al. (2007) found that comfrey contributed to the antiinflammatory activity of the multi-herb equine product that they tested on pigs. Devil's claw (*Harpagophytum procumbens*) may be a safe and effective treatment option for arthritis (Brien et al., 2006). In their review paper Setty and Sigal (2005) conclude that willow bark extract (*Salix* spp.) and nettles (*Urtica dioica*) are effective treatments for osteoarthritis. Sarsaparilla (*Smilax officinalis*) may be useful in the long-term treatment of clinical rheumatoid arthritis (Jiang and Xu et al., 2003; Shao et al., 2007). The safety of black walnut (*Juglans nigra*) and comfrey (*Symphytum officinale*) root extract (used externally) to treat osteoarthritis in pets should be investigated.

References

Ahmad, S.F., Khan, B., Bani, S., Suri, K.A., Satti, N.K., Qazi, G.N. 2006. Amelioration of adjuvant-induced arthritis by ursolic acid through altered Th1/Th2 cytokine production. Pharmacological Research 53, 233-40.

Ahmed, S., Anuntiyo, J., Malemud, C.J., Haqqi, T.M. 2005. Biological basis for the use of botanicals in osteoarthritis and rheumatoid arthritis: A review. *Evidence Based* Complementary and Alternative Medicine 2, 301-8.

Alves, D.S., Perez-Fons, L., Estepa, A., Micol, V. 2004. Membrane-related effects underlying the biological activity of the anthraquinones emodin and barbaloin. Biochemical Pharmacology 68, 549–561.

Anon, 2006. Monograph. *Eleutherococcus senticosus*. Alternative Medicine Review 11,151-5.

Anon, 2000. Berberine monograph. Alternative Medicine Review 5, 175-177.

Arts, I.C., Hollman, P.C. 2005. Polyphenols and disease risk in epidemiologic studies. The American Journal of Clinical Nutrition 81(1 Suppl), 317S-325S.

Ball, A.R., Casadei, G., Samosorn, S., Bremner, J.B., Ausubel, F.M., Moy, T.I., Lewis, K. 2006. Conjugating berberine to a multidrug efflux pump inhibitor creates an effective antimicrobial. ACS Chemical Biology 1, 594-600.

Banerjee, S,K, Maulik, S.K. 2002. Effect of garlic on cardiovascular disorders: A review. Nutrition Journal 1, 4.

Barrett, R., Zwickey, H. 2006. The effect of *Echinacea purpurea*, *Astragalus membranaceus* and *Glycyrrhiza glabra* on CD69 expression and immune cell activation in humans. Phytotherapy Research 20, 687-95.

Basch, E., Bent, S., Foppa, I., Haskmi, S., Kroll, D., Mele, M., Szapary, P., Ulbricht, C., Vora, M., Yong, S. 2006. Marigold (*Calendula officinalis* L.): An evidence-based systematic review by the Natural Standard Research Collaboration. Journal of Herbal Pharmacotherapy 6,135-59.

Brien, S., Lewith, G.T., McGregor, G. 2006. Devil's Claw (*Harpagophytum procumbens*) as a treatment for osteoarthritis: A review of efficacy and safety. Journal of Alternative and Complementary Medicine 12, 981-93.

Brush, J., Mendenhall, E., Guggenheim, A., Chan, T., Connelly, E., Soumyanath, A., Buresh, R., Barrett, R., Zwickey, H. 2006. The effect of *Echinacea purpurea*, *Astragalus membranaceus* and *Glycyrrhiza glabra* on CD69 expression and immune cell activation in humans. Phytotherapy Research 20, 687-95.

Burdette, J.E., Liu, J., Chen, S.N., Fabricant, D.S., Piersen, C.E., Barker, E.L., Pezzuto, J.M., Mesecar, A., Van Breemen, R.B., Farnsworth, N.R., Bolton, J.L. 2003. Black cohosh acts as a mixed competitive ligand and partial agonist of the serotonin receptor. Journal of Agricultural and Food Chemistry 51, 5661-70.

Caldefie-Chezet, F., Fusillier, C., Jarde, T., Laroye, H., Damez, M., Vasson, M.P., Guillot, J. 2006. Potential anti-inflammatory effects of *Melaleuca alternifolia* essential oil on human peripheral blood leukocytes. Phytotherapy Research 20, 364-370.

Cansaran, D., Kahya, D., Yurdakulola, E., Atakol, O.2006. Identification and quantitation of usnic acid from the lichen *Usnea* species of Anatolia and antimicrobial activity. Zeitschrift für Naturforschung. C, Journal of Biosciences 61, 773-6.

Cech, N.B., Tutor, K., Doty, B.A., Spelman, K., Sasagawa, M., Raner, G.M., Wenner, C.A. 2006. Liver enzyme-mediated oxidation of *Echinacea purpurea* alkylamides: Production of novel metabolites and changes in immunomodulatory activity. Planta Medica 72, 1372-7.

Chen, C.S., Chen, N.J., Lin, L.W., Hsieh, C.C., Chen, G.W., Hsieh, M.T.2006. Effects of Scutellariae Radix on gene expression in HEK 293 cells using cDNA microarray. Journal of Ethnopharmacology 105, 346-51.

Chiang, L.C., Chiang, W., Chang, M.Y., Lin, C.C. 2003. *In vitro* cytotoxic, antiviral and immunomodulatory effects of *Plantago major* and *Plantago asiatica*. American Journal of Chinese Medicine 31, 225-34.

Cho, E.J., Yokozawa, T., Rhyu, D.Y., Kim, H.Y., Shibahara, N., Park, J.C.2003. The inhibitory effects of 12 medicinal plants and their component compounds on lipid peroxidation. American Journal of Chinese Medicine 31 ,907-17.

Cho, M.K., Jang, Y.P., Kim, Y.C., Kim, S.G. 2004. Arctigenin, a phenylpropanoid dibenzylbutyrolactone lignan, inhibits MAP kinases and AP-1 activation via potent MKK inhibition: the role in TNF-alpha inhibition. International Immunopharmacology 4,1419-29.

Choi, E.M., Hwang, J.K.2005. Effect of some medicinal plants on plasma antioxidant system and lipid levels in rats. Phytotherapy Research 19 ,382-6.

Chrubasik, J.E., Roufogalis, B.D., Wagner, H., Chrubasik, S.A. 2007. A comprehensive review on nettle effect and efficacy profiles, Part I: Herba urticae. Phytomedicine 14 ,423-35.

Colvard, M.D., Cordell, G.A., Villalobos, R., Sancho, G., Soejarto, D.D., Pestle, W., Echeverri, T.L., Perkowitz, K.M., Michel, J. 2006. Survey of medical ethnobotanicals for dental and oral medicine conditions and pathologies. Journal of Ethnopharmacology 107,134–142.

Culver, C.A., Michalowski, S.M., Maia, R.C., Laster, S.M. 2005. The anti-apoptotic effects of nordihydroguaiaretic acid: inhibition of cPLA(2) activation during TNF-induced apoptosis arises from inhibition of calcium signaling. Life Sciences 77, 2457-70.

D'Anjou, M.A., Moreau, M., Troncy, E., Martel-Pelletier, J., Abram, F., Raynauld, J.P., Pelletier, J.P.2008. Osteophytosis, subchondral bone sclerosis, joint effusion and soft tissue thickening in canine experimental stifle osteoarthritis: Comparison between 1.5 T magnetic resonance imaging and computed radiography. Veterinary Surgery 37,166-77.

Dattner, A.M. 2003. From medical herbalism to phytotherapy in dermatology: Back to the future. Dermatologic Therapy 16,106-113.

de Almeida, R.N., Motta, S.C., de Brito Faturi, C., Catallani, B., Leite, J.R. 2004. Anxiolytic-like effects of rose oil inhalation on the elevated plus-maze test in rats. Pharmacology, Biochemistry, and Behaviour 77,361-4.

Di, D.L., Liu, Y.W., Ma, Z.G., Jiang, S.X. 2003. Determination of four alkaloids in *Berberis* plants by HPLC. Zhongguo Zhong Yao Za Zhi 28 ,1132-4.

Duke, J. A. 2008. Phytochemical and Ethnobotanical Databases. USDA-ARS-NGRL, Beltsville Agricultural Research Center, Beltsville, Maryland, USA.

Ebringerova, A., Kardosova, A., Hromadkova, Z., Hribalova, V. 2003. Mitogenic and comitogenic activities of polysaccharides from some European herbaceous plants. Fitoterapia 74,52-61.

Erdemoglu, N., Kupeli, E., Yesilada, E.2003. Anti-inflammatory and antinociceptive activity assessment of plants used as remedy in Turkish folk medicine. Journal of Ethnopharmacology 89,123-9.

Fiebich, B.L., Chrubasik, S. 2004. Effects of an ethanolic Salix extract on the release of selected inflammatory mediators *in vitro*. Phytomedicine 11(2-3),135-8.

Gagnier, J.J., van Tulder, M.W., Berman, B., Bombardier, C. 2007. Herbal medicine for low back pain. Cochrane Database of Systematic Reviews 32 , 82–92.

Gao, J., Huang, F., Zhang, Zhu, G., Yang, M., Xiao, P.2006. Cytotoxic cycloartane triterpene saponins from *Actaea asiatica*. Journal of Natural Products 69,1500-1502.

Garbutt, F., Jenner, R. 2004. Best evidence topic report. Wound closure in animal bites. Emerg Med J. 21 ,589-90.

Gershwin, L.J. 2007. Veterinary autoimmunity: Autoimmune diseases in domestic animals. Annals of the New York Academy of Science 1109,109-16.

Gorchakova, T.V., Suprun, I.V., Sobenin, I.A., Orekhov, A.N.2007. Use of natural products in anticytokine therapy. Bulletin of Experimental Biology and Medicine 143 ,316-9.

Gregory, P.J., Sperry, M., Wilson, A.F.2008. Dietary supplements for osteoarthritis. American Family Physician 77,177-84.

Grube, B., Grunwald, J., Krug, L., Staiger, C.2007. Efficacy of a comfrey root (Symphyti offic. radix) extract ointment in the treatment of patients with painful osteoarthritis of the knee: Results of a double-blind, randomised, bicenter, placebo-controlled trial. Phytomedicine 14,2-10.

Gundermann, K.J., Müller, J. 2007. Phytodolor--effects and efficacy of a herbal medicine. Wiener Medizinische Wochenschrift 157(13-14),343-7.

Hajhashemi, V., Ghannadi, A., Sharif, B. 2003. Anti-inflammatory and analgesic properties of the leaf extracts and essential oil of *Lavandula angustifolia* Mill. Journal of Ethnopharmacology 89 , 67-71.

Halcon, L., Milkus, K. 2004. *Staphylococcus aureus* and wounds: A review of tea tree oil as a promising antimicrobial. American Journal of Infection Control 32 ,402-8.

Hausmann, M., Obermeier, F., Paper, D.H., Balan, K., Dunger, N., Menzel, K., Falk, W., Schoelmerich, J., Herfarth, H., Rogler, G. 2007. *In vivo* treatment with the herbal phenylethanoid acteoside ameliorates intestinal inflammation in dextran sulphate sodium-induced colitis. Clinical and Experimental Immunology 148,373-81.

Hashidoko, Y. 1996. The phytochemistry of *Rosa rugosa*. Phytochemistry 43, 535-549.

Hegemann, N., Wondimu, A., Ullrich, K., Schmidt, M.F. 2003. Synovial MMP-3 and TIMP-1 levels and their correlation with cytokine expression in canine rheumatoid arthritis. Veterinary Immunology and Immunopathology 91(3-4),199-204.

Henrotin, Y., Sanchez, C., Balligand, M. 2005. Pharmaceutical and nutraceutical management of canine osteoarthritis: Present and future perspectives. Veterinary Journal 170,113-23.

Henrotin, Y. 2006. Nutraceuticals in the management of osteoarthritis: an overview. Journal of Veterinary Pharmacology and Therapeutics 29 Suppl 1,201.

Heron, S., Yarnell, E. 2001. The safety of low-dose *Larrea tridentata* (DC) Coville (creosote bush or chaparral): A retrospective clinical study. Journal of Alternative and Complementary Medicine 7,175-85.

Hsieh, C.J., Hall, K., Ha, T., Li, C., Krishnaswamy, G., Chi, D.S. 2007. Baicalein inhibits IL-1beta- and TNF-alpha-induced inflammatory cytokine production from human mast cells via regulation of the NF-kappaB pathway. Clinical and Molecular Allergy 5,5.

Hur, Y.G., Suh, C.H., Kim, S., Won, J. 2007. Rosmarinic acid induces apoptosis of activated T cells from rheumatoid arthritis patients via mitochondrial pathway. The Journal of Allergy and Clinical Immunology 27,36-45.

Jiang, J., Xu, Q. 2003. Immunomodulatory activity of the aqueous extract from rhizome of *Smilax glabra* in the later phase of adjuvant-induced arthritis in rats. Journal of Ethnopharmacology 85, 53-9.

Jiao, Y.B., Rui, Y.C., Yang, P.Y., Li, T.J., Qiu, Y. 2007. Effects of *Ginkgo biloba* extract on expressions of IL-1beta, TNF-alpha, and IL-10 in U937 foam cells. Yao Xue Xue Bao 42 ,930-4.

Ji, L.L., Laya, D., Chung, E., Fua, Y., Peterson, D.M. 2003. Effects of avenanthramides on oxidant generation and antioxidant enzyme activity in exercised rats. Nutrition Research 23, 1579–1590.

Juhás, S., Cikos, S., Czikková, S., Veselá, J., Il'ková, G., Hájek, T., Domaracká, K., Domaracký, M., Bujnáková, D., Rehák, P., Koppel, J. 2008. Effects of borneol and thymoquinone on TNBS-induced colitis in mice. Folia Biologica (Praha). 54,1-7.

Jung, Y.B., Roh, K.J., Jung, J.A., Jung, K., Yoo, H., Cho, Y.B., Kwak, W.J., Kim, D.K., Kim, K.H., Han, C.K. 2001. Effect of SKI 306X, a new herbal anti-arthritic agent, in patients with osteoarthritis of the knee: A double-blind placebo controlled study. American Journal of Chinese Medicine 29(3-4), 485-91.

Kaji, K., Yoshida, S., Nagata, N., Yamashita, T., Mizukoshi, E., Honda, M., Kojima, Y., Kaneko, S. 2004. An open-label study of administration of EH0202, a health-food additive, to patients with chronic hepatitis C. Journal of Gastroenterology 39, 873-8.

Khanna, D., Sethi, G., Ahn, K.S., Pandey, M.K., Kunnumakkara, A.B., Sung, B., Aggarwal, A., Aggarwal, B.B.2007. Natural products as a gold mine for arthritis treatment. Current Opinion in Pharmacology 7, 344-51.

Kisiel, W., Zielińska, K. 2000. Sesquiterpenoids and phenolics from *Lactuca perennis*. Fitoterapia 71, 86-87.

Kormosh, N., Laktionov, K., Antoshechkina, M. 2006. Effect of a combination of extract from several plants on cell-mediated and humoral immunity of patients with advanced ovarian cancer. Phytotherapy Research 20 ,424-5.

Kumarasamy, Y., Cox, P.J., Jaspars, M., Nahar, L., Sarker, S.D. 2002. Screening seeds of Scottish plants for antibacterial activity. Journal of Ethnopharmacology 83(1-2),73-7.

Kwon, K.H., Murakami, A., Tanaka, T., Ohigashi, H. 2005. Dietary rutin, but not its aglycone quercetin, ameliorates dextran sulfate sodium-induced experimental colitis in mice: attenuation of pro-inflammatory gene expression. Biochemical Pharmacology 69 ,395-406.

Lajeunesse, D., Reboul, P. 2003. Subchondral bone in osteoarthritis: A biologic link with articular cartilage leading to abnormal remodeling. Current Opinion in Rheumatology 15 ,628-33.

Kaszkin, M., Beck, K.F., Koch, E., Erdelmeier, C., Kusch, S., Pfeilschifter, J., Loew, D. 2004. Downregulation of iNOS expression in rat mesangial cells by special extracts of *Harpagophytum procumbens* derives from harpagoside-dependent and independent effects. Phytomedicine 11(7-8),585-95.

Keiss, H.P., Dirsch, V.M., Hartung, T., Haffner, T., Trueman, L., Auger, J., Kahane, R., Vollmar, A.M. 2003. Garlic (*Allium sativum* L.) modulates cytokine expression in lipopolysaccharide-activated human blood thereby inhibiting NF-kappaB activity. The Journal of Nutrition 133,2171-5.

Kim, C.D., Lee, W.K., Lee, M.H., Cho, H.S., Lee, Y.K., Roh, S.S. 2004. Inhibition of mast cell-dependent allergy reaction by extract of black cohosh (*Cimicifuga racemosa*). Immunopharmacology and Immunotoxicology 26,299-308.

Kim, M.H., Joo, H.G. 2008. Immunostimulatory effects of fucoidan on bone marrow-derived dendritic cells. Immunology Letters 115,138-43.

Küpeli, E., Koşar, M., Yeşilada, E., Hüsnü, K., Başer, C. 2002. A comparative study on the anti-inflammatory, antinociceptive and antipyretic effects of isoquinoline alkaloids from the roots of Turkish Berberis species. Life Sciences 72, 645-57.

Kwon, K.H., Murakami, A., Ohigashi, H. 2004. Suppressive effects of natural and synthetic agents on dextran sulfate sodium-induced interleukin-1beta release from murine peritoneal macrophages. Bioscience, Biotechnology, and Biochemistry 68,436-9.

Kyung, T.W., Lee, J.E., Shin, H.H., Choi, H.S. 2008. Rutin inhibits osteoclast formation by decreasing reactive oxygen species and TNF-alpha by inhibiting activation of NF-kappaB. Experimental and Molecular Medicine 40,52-8.

Lans, C., Turner, N., Brauer, G., Lourenco, G., Georges, K. 2006. Ethnoveterinary medicines used for horses in Trinidad and in British Columbia, Canada. Journal of Ethnobiology and Ethnomedicine 2,31.

Lemburg, A.K., Meyer-Lindenberg, A., Hewicker-Trautwein, M. 2004. Immunohistochemical characterization of inflammatory cell populations and adhesion molecule expression in synovial membranes from dogs with spontaneous cranial cruciate ligament rupture. Veterinary Immunology and Immunopathology 97(3-4),231-40.

Li, J.X., Yu, Z.Y.2006. Cimicifugae rhizoma: from origins, bioactive constituents to clinical outcomes. Current Medicinal Chemistry 13(24),2927-51.

Lin, F.Y., Chen, Y.H., Chen, Y.L., Wu, T.C., Li, C.Y., Chen, J.W., Lin, S.J.2007. *Ginkgo biloba* extract inhibits endotoxin-induced human aortic smooth muscle cell proliferation via suppression of toll-like receptor 4 expression and NADPH oxidase activation. Journal of Agricultural and Food Chemistry 55 ,1977-84.

Liu, L., Zubik, L., Collins, F.W., Marko, M., Meydani, M. 2004a. The antiatherogenic potential of oat phenolic compounds. Atherosclerosis 175,39-49.

Liu, Z-F., Fang, F., Dong, Y-S., Li, G., Zhen, H. 2004. Experimental study on the prevention and treatment of murine cytomegalovirus hepatitis by using allitridin. Antiviral Research 61,125–128.

Lohmann, Klaus, Reininger Eveline, Bauer, Rudolf. 2000. Screening of European anti-inflammatory herbal drugs for inhibition of cyclooxygenase 1 and 2. Phytomedicine, Supplement II: 99.

Lukaczer, D., Darland, G., Tripp, M., Liska, D., Lerman, R.H., Schiltz, B., Bland, J.S. 2005. A pilot trial evaluating Meta050, a proprietary combination of reduced iso-alpha acids, rosemary extract and oleanolic acid in patients with arthritis and fibromyalgia. Phytotherapy Research 9, 864-9.

Ma, Y., Wink, M. 2008. Lobeline, a piperidine alkaloid from Lobelia can reverse P-gp dependent multidrug resistance in tumor cells. Phytomedicine 15(9):754-8

Mamani-Matsuda, M., Kauss, T., Al-Kharrat, A., Rambert, J., Fawaz, F., Thiolat, D., Moynet, D., Coves, S., Malvy, D., Mossalayi, M.D. 2006. Therapeutic and preventive properties of quercetin in experimental arthritis correlate with decreased macrophage inflammatory mediators. Biochemical Pharmacology 72 ,1304-10.

Matsuda, H., Wang, Q., Matsuhira, K., Nakamura, S., Yuan, D., Yoshikawa, M. 2008. Inhibitory effects of thunberginols A and B isolated from Hydrangeae Dulcis Folium on mRNA expression of cytokines and on activation of activator protein-1 in RBL-2H3 cells. Phytomedicine 15,177-84.

Maoka, T.., Mochida, K., Kozuka, M., Ito, Y., Fujiwara, Y., Hashimoto. K., Enjo, F., Ogata, M., Nobukuni, Y., Tokuda, H., Nishino, H. 2001. Cancer chemopreventive activity of carotenoids in the fruits of red paprika *Capsicum annuum* L. Cancer Letters 172, 103–109.

Meckes, M., David-Rivera, A.D., Nava-Aguilar, V., Jimenez, A. 2004. Activity of some Mexican medicinal plant extracts on carrageenan-induced rat paw edema. Phytomedicine 11 ,446-51.

Mekhfi, H., El Haouari, M., Legssyer, A., Bnouham, M., Aziz, M., Atmani, F., Remmal, A., Ziyyat, A. 2004. Platelet anti-aggregant property of some Moroccan medicinal plants. Journal of Ethnopharmacology 94(2-3),317-22.

Mix, J., Crews, D. 2000. An examination of the efficacy of *Ginkgo biloba* extract EGb 761 on the neuropsychologic functioning of cognitively intact older adults. Journal of Alternative and Complement Medicine 6,219-29.

Morita, H., Iizuka, T., Choo, C.Y., Chan, K.L., Itokawa, H., Takeya, K. 2005. Dichotomins J and K, vasodilator cyclic peptides from *Stellaria dichotoma*. Journal of Natural Products 68 ,1686-8.

Muir, P., Schaefer, S.L., Manley, P.A., Svaren, J.P., Oldenhoff, W.E., Hao, Z. 2007. Expression of immune response genes in the stifle joint of dogs with oligoarthritis and degenerative cranial cruciate ligament rupture. Veterinary Immunology and Immunopathology 119(3-4),214-21.

Nam, J.H., Jung, H.J., Choi, J., Lee, K.T., Park, H.J.2006. The anti-gastropathic and anti-rheumatic effect of niga-ichigoside F1 and 23-hydroxytormentic acid isolated from the unripe fruits of *Rubus coreanus* in a rat model. Biological & Pharmaceutical Bulletin 29 ,967-70.

Nie, L., Wise, M.L., Peterson, D.M., Meydani, M. 2006. Avenanthramide, a polyphenol from oats, inhibits vascular smooth muscle cell proliferation and enhances nitric oxide production. Atherosclerosis 186, 260–266.

Noli, C., Miolo, A. 2001. The mast cell in wound healing. Vet Dermatol. 12 ,303-13.

Nuntanakorn, P., Jiang, B., Einbond, L.S., Yang, H., Kronenberg, F., Weinstein, B., Kennelly, E.J. 2006. Polyphenolic constituents of *Actaea racemosa*. Journal of Natural Products 69, 314-318.

Papoutsi, Z., Kassi, E., Chinou, I., Halabalaki, M., Skaltsounis, L.A., Moutsatsou, P. 2008. Walnut extract (*Juglans regia* L.) and its component ellagic acid exhibit anti-inflammatory activity in human aorta endothelial cells and osteoblastic activity in the cell line KS483. Br Journal of Nutrition 99 ,715-22.

Park, S.Y., Hong, S.S., Han, X.H., Hwang, J.S., Lee, D., Ro, J.S., Hwang, B.Y.2007. Lignans from *Arctium lappa* and their inhibition of LPS-induced nitric oxide production. Chemical & Pharmaceutical Bulletin (Tokyo). 55,150-2.

Pearson, W., Orth, M.W., Lindinger, M.I. 2007. Differential anti-inflammatory and chondroprotective effects of simulated digests of indomethacin and an herbal composite (Mobility) in a cartilage explant model of articular inflammation. Journal of Veterinary Pharmacology and Therapeutics 30 ,523-33.

Pereira, L.M., Hatanaka, E., Martins, E.F., Oliveira, F., Liberti, E.A., Farsky, S.H., Curi, R., Pithon-Curi, T.C. 2008. Effect of oleic and linoleic acids on the inflammatory phase of wound healing in rats. Cell Biochemistry and Function 26,197-204.

Philipov, S., Istatkova, R., Ivanovska, N., Denkova, P., Tosheva, K., Navas, H., Villegas, J. 1998. Phytochemical study and antiinflammatory properties of *Lobelia laxiflora* L. Zeitschrift für Naturforschung. C, Journal of Biosciences. 53(5-6),311-7.

Pommier, P., Gomez, F., Sunyach, M.P., D'Hombres, A., Carrie, C., Montbarbon, X. 2004. Phase III randomized trial of *Calendula officinalis* compared with trolamine for the prevention of acute dermatitis during irradiation for breast cancer. American Journal of Clinical Oncology 22 ,1447-1453.

Psotová, J., Kolář, M., Soušek J., Švagera Z., Vičar, J., Ulrichová Jitka. 2003. Biological activities of *Prunella vulgaris* extract. Phytotherapy Research 17 ,1082-7.

Psotová, J., Chlopcíková, S., Miketová, P., Hrbác, J., Simánek, V. 2004. Chemoprotective effect of plant phenolics against anthracycline-induced toxicity on rat cardiomyocytes. Part III. Apigenin, baicalelin, kaempherol, luteolin and quercetin. Phytotherapy Research 18 ,516-21.

Qiu, S.X., Dan, C., Ding, L.S., Peng, S., Chen, S.N., Farnsworth, N.R., Nolta, J., Gross, M.L., Zhou, P. 2007. A triterpene glycoside from black cohosh that inhibits osteoclastogenesis by modulating RANKL and TNFalpha signaling pathways. ACS Chemical Biology 14 ,860-9.

Raghavenra, H., Diwakr, B.T., Lokesh, B.R., Naidu, K.A. 2006. Eugenol--the active principle from cloves inhibits 5-lipoxygenase activity and leukotriene-C4 in human PMNL cells. Prostaglandins, Leukotrienes, and Essential Fatty Acids 74,23-7.

Rhyu, M.R., Lu, J., Webster, D.E., Fabricant, D.S., Farnsworth, N.R., Wang, Z.J. 2006. Black cohosh (*Actaea racemosa, Cimicifuga racemosa*) behaves as a mixed competitive ligand and partial agonist at the human mu opiate receptor. Journal of Agricultural and Food Chemistry 54(26),9852-7.

Rossetti, R.G., Seiler, C.M., DeLuca, P., Laposata, M., Zurier, R.B. 1997. Oral administration of unsaturated fatty acids: effects on human peripheral blood T lymphocyte proliferation. Journal of Leukocyte Biology 62 ,438-43.

Rotelli, A.E., Guardia, T., Juárez, A.O., de la Rocha, N.E., Pelzer, L.E. 2003. Comparative study of flavonoids in experimental models of inflammation. Pharmacological Research 48 ,601-6.

Roy, J., Messier, S., Labrecque, O., Cox, W.R. 2007. Clinical and *in vitro* efficacy of amoxicillin against bacteria associated with feline skin wounds and abscesses. Can Veterinary Journal 48 ,607-11.

Ruperez, P., Ahrazem, O., Leal, J.A. 2002. Potential antioxidant capacity of sulfated polysaccharides from the edible marine brown seaweed *Fucus vesiculosus*. Journal of Agricultural and Food Chemistry 50 , 840-5.

Ryu, M., Kim, E.H., Chun, M., Kang, S., Shim, B., Yu, Y.B., Jeong, G., Lee, J.S. 2008. Astragali Radix elicits anti-inflammation via activation of MKP-1, concomitant with attenuation of p38 and Erk. Journal of Ethnopharmacology 115,184-93.

Schütz, K., Carle, R., Schieber, A. 2006. Taraxacum--A review on its phytochemical and pharmacological profile. Journal of Ethnopharmacology 107 ,313-23.

Schulze-Tanzil, G., De S.P., Behnke, B., Klingelhoefer, S., Scheid, A., Shakibaei, M. 2002. Effects of the antirheumatic remedy hox alpha--a new stinging nettle leaf extract--on matrix metalloproteinases in human chondrocytes *in vitro*. Histology and Histopathology 17,477-85.

Schulze-Tanzil, G., Hansen, C., Shakibaei, M. 2004. Effect of a *Harpagophytum procumbens* DC extract on matrix metalloproteinases in human chondrocytes *in vitro*. Arzneimittelforschung 54 ,213-20. Article in German.

Scrivo, R., Di Franco, M., Spadaro, A., Valesini, G. 2007. The immunology of rheumatoid arthritis. Annals of the New York Academy of Science 1108,312-22.

Setty, A.R., Sigal, L.H.2005. Herbal medications commonly used in the practice of rheumatology: Mechanisms of action, efficacy, and side effects. Seminars in Arthritis and Rheumatism 34 ,773-84.

Shao, B., Guo, H., Cui, Y., Ye, M., Han, J., Guo, D. 2007. Steroidal saponins from *Smilax china* and their anti-inflammatory activities. Phytochemistry 68 ,623-30.

Shetty, B.S., Udupa, S.L., Udupa, A.L., Somayaji, S.N. 2006. Effect of *Centella asiatica* L (Umbelliferae) on normal and dexamethasone-suppressed wound healing in Wistar Albino rats. The International Journal of Lower Extremity Wounds 5 ,137-43.

Shishodia, S., Majumdar, S., Banerjee, S., Aggarwal, B.B. 2003. Ursolic acid inhibits nuclear factor-kappaB activation induced by carcinogenic agents through suppression of IkappaBalpha kinase and p65 phosphorylation: Correlation with down-regulation of cyclooxygenase 2, matrix metalloproteinase 9, and cyclin D1. Cancer Research 63 ,4375-83.

Shon, Y.H., Nam, K.S. 2003. Protective effect of Astragali radix extract on interleukin 1beta-induced inflammation in human amnion. Phytotherapy Research 17 ,1016-20.

Son, Y.O., Lee, K.Y., Choi, K.C., Chung, Y., Kim, J.G., Jeon, Y.M., Jang, Y.S., Lee, J.C. 2004. Inhibitory effects of glycoprotein-120 (G-120) from *Ulmus davidiana* Nakai on cell growth and activation of matrix metalloproteinases. Mol Cells. 18,163-70.

Subarnas, A., Tadano, T., Oshima, Y., Kisara, K., Ohizumi, Y. 1993. Pharmacological properties of beta-amyrin palmitate, a novel centrally acting compound, isolated from *Lobelia inflata* leaves. The Journal of Pharmacy and Pharmacology 45 ,545-50.

TAHCC, 2004. Alternative Animal Health Care in British Columbia: A manual of traditional practices used by herbalists, veterinarian, farmers and animal caretakers. The Traditional Animal Health Care Collaborative. Victoria, British Columbia, Canada.

Tipton, D.A., Lyle, B., Babich, H., Dabbous, M.K.h. 2003. *In vitro* cytotoxic and anti-inflammatory effects of myrrh oil on human gingival fibroblasts and epithelial cells. In vitro & Molecular Toxicology 17 ,301-10.

Tunón, H., Olavsdotter, C., Bohlin, L. 1995. Evaluation of anti-inflammatory activity of some Swedish medicinal plants. Inhibition of prostaglandin biosynthesis andPAF-induced exocytosis. Journal of Ethnopharmacology 48, 61-76.

Vermani, K., Garg, S., 2002. Herbal medicines for sexually transmitted diseases and AIDS. Journal of Ethnopharmacology 80, 49-66.

Wang, Q., Matsuda, H., Matsuhira, K., Nakamura, S., Yuan, D., Yoshikawa, M. 2007. Inhibitory effects of thunberginols A, B, and F on degranulations and releases of TNF-alpha and IL-4 in RBL-2H3 cells. Biological & Pharmaceutical Bulletin 30,388-92.

Westra, J., Brouwer, E., Bos, R., Posthumus, M.D., Doornbos-van der Meer, B., Kallenberg, C.G., Limburg, P.C. 2007. Regulation of cytokine-induced HIF-1alpha expression in rheumatoid synovial fibroblasts. Annals of the New York Academy of Science 1108,340-8.

Xie, J.Y., Dong, J.C., Gong, Z.H. 2006. Effects on herba epimedii and radix Astragali on tumor necrosis factor-alpha and nuclear factor-kappa B in asthmatic rats. Zhongguo Zhong Xi Yi Jie He Za Zhi 26 ,723-7. Article in Chinese.

Yildirim, A., Mavi, A., Kara, A.A. 2001. Determination of antioxidant and antimicrobial activities of *Rumex crispus* L. extracts. Journal of Agricultural and Food Chemistry 49 ,4083-9.

Youn, J., Lee, K.H., Won, J., Huh, S.J., Yun, H.S., Cho, W.G., Paik, D.J. 2003. Beneficial effects of rosmarinic acid on suppression of collagen induced arthritis. The Journal of Rheumatology 30 ,1203-7.

Zhao, W.S., Zhang, Y.Q., Ren, L.J., Zhang, L., Yang, J. 1993. Immunopotentiating effects of polysaccharides isolated from *Medicago sativa* L. Zhongguo Yao Li Xue Bao 14 ,273-6. Article in Chinese.

Zhai, Z., Liu, Y., Wu, L., Senchina, D.S., Wurtele, E.S., Murphy, P.A., Kohut, M.L., Cunnick, J.E. 2007. Enhancement of innate and adaptive immune functions by multiple *Echinacea* species. Journal of Medicinal Food 10 ,423-34.

Zhang WJ, Hufnagl P, Binder BR, Wojta J. 2003. Antiinflammatory activity of astragaloside IV is mediated by inhibition of NF-kappaB activation and adhesion molecule expression. Journal of Thrombosis and Haemostasis 90 ,904-14.

Zheng, W., Wang, S.Y. 2001. Antioxidant activity and phenolic compounds in selected herbs. Journal of Agricultural and Food Chemistry 49 ,5165-70.

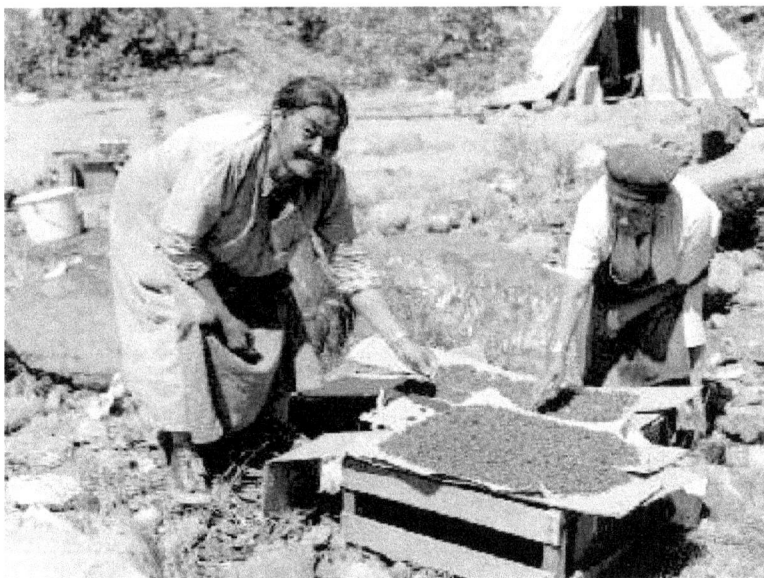

"Lillooet Indians drying berries," 1954.

Photo: British Columbia Archives

TABLE 2. ETHNOVETERINARY PLANTS USED FOR INJURIES AND ANAL GLAND PROBLEMS IN PETS IN BRITISH COLUMBIA

Scientific name	Common name	Plant part used	Use
Allium sativum L. (Alliaceae)	garlic	clove	swollen anal gland
Aloe vera. L. (Liliaceae)	aloe	gel	external treatment for swollen anal gland
Astragalus membranaceus (Fisch.) (Fabaceae)	astragalus	root	dog bite
Avena sativa L. (Poaceae)	oatstraw	tincture	comatose raccoon
Calendula L. (Asteraceae)	calendula	flower	gum inflammation from broken tooth, dog bites, wounds, sprains, post-operative bleeding, anal gland problems
Commiphora molmol Engl. (Burseraceae)	myrrh	resin, oil	bleeding wounds, sprains, post-operative bleeding, deep wounds, abrasions, gum inflammation from broken tooth
Eleutherococcus senticosus Rupr. & Maxim.) Maxim. (Araliaceae)	eleuthero	tincture	comatose raccoon
Echinacea Moench (Asteraceae)	Echinacea	root	snakebites, dog bites, wounds
Fagus sylvatica L. (Fagaceae)	beech	tincture	comatose raccoon
Ginkgo biloba L. (Ginkgoaceae)	ginkgo	tincture	comatose raccoon
Hydocotyle asiatica/ Centella asiatica L. (Apiaceae)	gotu kola	tincture	comatose raccoon
Hydrastis canadensis L. (Ranunculaceae)	goldenseal	leaves	dog bites, bleeding wounds, sprains, post-operative bleeding, deep wounds, abrasions
Hypericum perforatum L. (Hypericaceae)	St. John's wort	flowers	skin conditions, sprains, post-operative bleeding, deep wounds, abrasions, surgery scars, comatose raccoon
Lavandula officinalis L. (Labiatae)	lavender	flowers	wounds, sprains, post-operative bleeding, abrasions

TABLE 3. ETHNOVETERINARY PLANTS USED FOR INJURIESAND ANAL GLAND PROBLEMS IN PETS IN BRITISH COLUMBIA

Scientific name	Common name	Plant part used	Use
Berberis aquifolium Pursh./ *Mahonia aquifolium* (Berberidaceae)	Oregon grape	root	wounds, sprains, post-operative bleeding, abrasions
Medicago sativa L. (Fabaceae)	alfalfa	tincture	comatose raccoon
Melaleuca alternifolia L. (Myrtaceae)	tea tree	oil	wounds, sprains, post-operative bleeding, abrasions
Origanum vulgare L. (Labiatae)	oregano	leaves	wounds, sprains, post-operative bleeding, abrasions
Plantago major L. (Plantaginaceae)	plantain	leaves	snake bite, wounds, sprains, post-operative bleeding, abscesses, anal gland problems
Prunella vulgaris L. (Lamiaceae)	all-heal/self heal	flowering tops	wounds, sprains, post-operative bleeding, abrasions
Rosa gymnocarpa Nutt. (Rosaceae)	rose	hips	gum inflammation from broken tooth
Rubus idaeus L., *Rubus* spp. (Rosaceae)	raspberry	leaves	wounds, sprains, post-op bleeding, abrasions
Rumex crispus L. (Polygonaceae)	yellow dock	leaves	snake bite
Salvia officinalis L. (Lamiaceae)	sage	aerial parts	gum inflammation from broken tooth
Scutellaria lateriflora L. (Lamiaceae)	skullcap	tincture	comatose raccoon
Stellaria media (L.) Cyrill. (Caryophyllaceae)	chickweed	aerial parts	wounds, sprains, post-op bleeding, abrasions
Symphytum officinale L. (Boraginaceae)	comfrey	leaves, roots	dog bites, bleeding wounds, sprains, post-operative bleeding, deep wounds, abrasions
Ulmus fulva Michx. (Ulmaceae)	slippery elm	bark	wounds, sprains, post-op bleeding, abrasions, swollen anal gland
Urtica dioica L. (Urticaceae)	nettles	plant tops	wounds, sprains, post-op bleeding, abrasions, swollen anal gland
Usnea longissima Ach. (Parmeliaceae)	usnea	whole lichen	anal gland problems

TABLE 4. ETHNOVETERINARY REMEDIES IN BRITISH COLUMBIA FOR PETS FOR RHEUMATOID ARTHRITIS JOINT PAIN AND ARTICULAR CARTILAGE INJURIES

Scientific name	Common name	Plant part used	Use
Actea/Cimicifuga racemosa (L.) Nutt., (Ranunculaceae)	black cohosh	root	rheumatoid arthritis, joint pain
Allium sativum L. (Alliaceae)	garlic	clove	articular cartilage injury
Arctium lappa L. (Asteraceae)	burdock	root	rheumatoid arthritis, joint pain
Capsicum spp. (Solanaceae)	cayenne	powder	arthritis, bruising, rheumatoid arthritis
Equisetum palustre L. (Equisetaceae)	horsetail	aerial parts	arthritis, bruising, rheumatoid arthritis
Fucus vesiculosus L. (Fucaceae; Brown Algae)	kelp	whole	articular cartilage injury
Harpagophytum procumbens DC (Pedaliaceae)	devil's claw	roots	rheumatoid arthritis, joint pain
Hydrangea arborescens L. (Hydrangeaceae)	hydrangea	root	rheumatoid arthritis, joint pain
Juglans nigra L. (Juglandaceae)	black walnut	fruit hull	rheumatoid arthritis, joint pain
Lactuca muralis (L.) P. Gaertn. (Asteraceae)	wild lettuce	leaves	rheumatoid arthritis, joint pain
Larrea tridentata (Sessé & Moc. ex DC.) Coville var. arenaria L. Benson (Zygophyllaceae)	chaparral	leaves	rheumatoid arthritis, joint pain
Lobelia inflata L. (Campanulaceae)	lobelia	aerial part	rheumatoid arthritis, joint pain
Medicago sativa L. (Fabaceae)	alfalfa	leaves	rheumatoid arthritis, joint pain, articular cartilage injury
Salix lucida Muhl. (Salicaceae)	white willow	bark	articular cartilage injury
Smilax officinalis L. (Smilacaceae)	sarsaparilla	root	rheumatoid arthritis, joint pain
Symphytum officinale L. (Boraginaceae)	comfrey	leaves & root	articular cartilage injury, partial tear of cruciate ligament
Taraxacum officinale Weber (Asteraceae)	dandelions	leaves & root	articular cartilage injury
Urtica dioica L. (Urticaceae)	stinging nettle	leaves	rheumatoid arthritis, joint pain. articular cartilage injury

TABLE 5. NON EXPERIMENTAL VALIDATION OF PLANTS USED FOR INJURIES AND OTHER PROBLEMS IN PETS IN BRITISH COLUMBIA.

Medicinal plant	Validation information	Reference	Validation
Actea/Cimicifuga racemosa	Ethnoveterinary use - rheumatoid arthritis, joint pain Black cohosh has several biological activities including antiinflammatory and vasoactive activities. Black cohosh has no clinically relevant effect on CYP3A activity *in vivo*. The ethanol extract of black cohosh acted as a mixed competitive ligand, displacing 77 +/- 4% [3H]DAMGO to hMOR (Ki = 62.9 microg/mL). *Actaea* species have 9,19-cycloartane triterpene glycosides.	Burdette et al., 2003; Li and Yu, 2006; Rhyu et al., 2006; Gao et al., 2006; Kim et al., 2004; Qiu et al., 2007	3
Allium sativum	Ethnoveterinary use -swollen anal gland, dietary supplement for articular cartilage injury Several favourable experimental and clinical effects of garlic preparations, including garlic extract are attributed to i) stimulation of immune function, ii) enhanced detoxification of foreign compounds, iii) antimicrobial effect and iv) antioxidant effect. *Allium sativum* can maintain immunologic homeostasis. Allitridin is responsible for garlic's antimicrobial and immunomodulatory activities and is currently used for the treatment of fungal and bacterial infections by intravenous infusion in China.	Banerjee and Maulik, 2002; Liu et al., 2004; Keiss et al., 2003	3
Aloe vera L. / *Aloe barbadensis*	Ethnoveterinary use -external treatment for swollen anal gland It is used for oral ulcers/inflammations and active compounds include anthracenes and carbohydrates. *Aloe vera* gels and aloins have dermatological applications	Colvard et al., 2006; Alves et al., 2004	4

	based on their capacity to inhibit the activity of microbial and human collagenases and metalloproteases.		
Arctium lappa	Ethnoveterinary use - rheumatoid arthritis, joint pain A new butyrolactone sesquilignan together with four known lignans, were isolated from the methanolic extract of the seeds from *Arctium lappa* plant. The two lignans, lappaol F and diarctigenin strongly inhibited NO production in the LPS-stimulated RAW264.7 cells with IC(50) values of 9.5 and 9.6 microM, respectively.	Park et al., 2007	2
Astragalus membranaceus	Ethnoveterinary use - dog bite *Echinacea purpurea, Astragalus membranaceus* and *Glycyrrhiza glabra* herbal tinctures stimulated immune cells as quantified by CD69 expression on CD4 and CD8 T cells in human subjects in a pilot study. This activation took place within 24 h of ingestion, and continued for at least 7 days. In addition, these three herbs had an additive effect on CD69 expression when used in combination.	Brush et al., 2006; Barrett and Zwickey, 2006; Ryu et al., 2008	3
Avena sativa	Ethnoveterinary use -raccoon in coma *Avena sativa* is used as a poultice or soak in folk medicine and is considered to be calming when taken internally. Studies have confirmed this anti-irritant property. Avenanthramides are polyphenols in oat kernels that help prevent atherosclerosis through inhibition of SMC proliferation and increasing NO production. They suppressed IL-1beta-stimulated expressions of intracellular adhesion molecule-1 (ICAM-1), vascular cell adhesion molecule-1	Dattner, 2003; Nie et al., 2006; Ji et al., 2003; Liu et al., 2004a	3

	(VCAM-1), and E-selectin and the secretion of proinflammatory cytokines IL-6, chemokines IL-8 and monocyte chemoattractant protein (MCP)-1. Other antioxidants found are tocotrienols, phenolic acids, flavonoids, sterols and phytic acid.		
Calendula officinalis	Ethnoveterinary use -abscesses, gum inflammation from broken tooth, anxiety associated with swollen anal gland, punctures, external treatment for swollen anal gland, dog bites, wounds, sprains, post-operative bleeding, external & internal treatment, burns *Calendula officinalis* can prevent acute dermatitis of grade 2 or higher and should be proposed for patients undergoing postoperative irradiation for breast cancer.	Pommier et al., 2004	3
Capsicum spp.	Ethnoveterinary use -arthritis, bruising, rheumatoid arthritis Three low-quality trials with *Capsicum frutescens* in topical preparations found good results against the control. Capsanthin and capsorubin have antioxidative activities.	Gagnier et al., 2006; Maoka et al., 2001	3
Commiphora molmol	Ethnoveterinary use -abscesses, bleeding wounds, sprains, post-operative bleeding, deep wounds, abrasions, gum inflammation from broken tooth, wounds, sprains, post-operative bleeding, abrasions Myrrh has antibacterial and anti-inflammatory activities. Myrrh oil (MO) had no 24 hour cytotoxicity to human gingival fibroblasts and epithelial cells. At 48 h, 0.0005-0.001% MO decreased epithelial cell viability 30-50%. At subtoxic MO levels (0.00001-0.001%), there was a significant reduction of IL-1beta-stimulated IL-6 and IL-8	Tipton et al., 2003	3

	production by fibroblasts, but not by epithelial cells.		
Echinacea purpurea	Ethnoveterinary use -snake bite, dog bites, wounds Echinacea compounds, the alkylamides, have immunomodulatory effects. Echinacea alkylamides suppressed IL-2 secretion by stimulated T cells, and this effect was significantly lessened upon oxidation of the alkylamides to carboxylic acids and hydroxylated metabolites.	Cech et al., 2006; Ball et al., 2006; Zhai et al., 2007	3
Eleutherococcus senticosus	Ethnoveterinary use -raccoon in coma A combination of dried ethanol/water extracts from roots of *Leuzea carthamoides*, *Rhodiola rosea*, *Eleutherococcus senticosus* and fruits of *Schizandra chinensis* (AdMax) was studied on twenty eight patients with stage III-IV epithelial ovarian cancer who were treated once with 75 mg/m(2) cisplatin and 600 mg/m(2) cyclophosphamide. In patients who took AdMax (270 mg a day) for 4 weeks following the chemotherapy, the mean numbers of the four T cell subclasses were increased in comparison with the mean numbers of the T cell subclasses in patients who did not take AdMax. In patients who took AdMax, the mean amounts of IgG and IgM were also increased. The combination of extracts from adaptogenic plants may boost the suppressed immunity in ovarian cancer patients undergoing chemotherapy.	Kormosh et al., 2006; Anon, 2006	3
Equisetum palustre	Ethnoveterinary use -arthritis, bruising, rheumatoid arthritis, abscesses *Equisetum arvense* extracts produced a	Mekhfi et al., 2004	2

	dose-dependent inhibition of thrombin and ADP-induced aggregation attributed to polyphenolic compounds.		
Fagus sylvatica	Ethnoveterinary use -raccoon in coma. No known clinical trials to evaluate.	No studies	
Fucus vesiculosus	Ethnoveterinary use -dietary supplement for articular cartilage injury Soluble fractions of the marine alga *Fucus vesiculosus* (42.3% yield) are composed of neutral sugars (18.9-48 g/100 g), uronic acids (8.8-52.8 g/100 g), sulfate (2.4-11.5 g/100 g), small amounts of protein (< 1-6.1 g/100 g), and nondialyzable polyphenols (0.1-2.7 g/100 g). The main neutral sugars were fucose, glucose, galactose, and xylose. Sulfated polysaccharides may be natural antioxidants. Fucoidan(polysaccharide) has immunostimulating effects.	Ruperez et al., 2002; Kim and Joo, 2008.	2
Ginkgo biloba	Ethnoveterinary use -raccoon in coma *Ginkgo biloba* extract is an anti-atherothrombotic Chinese herbal medicine with anti-inflammatory properties. Some clinical trials have demonstrated the efficacy of ginkgo extract in cognitively impaired persons. In the last decade ginkgo was approved as a treatment for dementia in Germany.	Lin et al., 2007; Mix and Crews, 2000; Jiao et al., 2007	3
Harpagophytum procumbens	Ethnoveterinary use - rheumatoid arthritis, joint pain Two high-quality trials utilizing *Harpagophytum procumbens* found strong evidence for short-term improvements in pain and rescue medication for daily doses standardized to 50 mg or 100 mg harpagoside with another high-quality trial demonstrating relative equivalence to 12.5 mg per day of rofecoxib, and it is safe	Gagnier et al., 2006; Brien et al., 2006	4

	(relative to NSAIDs).		
Hydocotyle asiatica/Centella asiatica	Ethnoveterinary use - raccoon in coma *Centella asiatica* extract significantly increased the wound breaking strength in an incision wound model compared to controls (P < .001). The extract-treated wounds were found to epithelize faster, and the rate of wound contraction was significantly increased as compared to control wounds (P < .001). The leaf extract promoted wound healing significantly and was able to overcome the wound-healing suppressing action of dexamethasone in a rat model.	Shetty et al., 2006	4
Hydrangea arborescens	Ethnoveterinary use - rheumatoid arthritis, joint pain Thunberginols A, B, and F from the processed leaves of *Hydrangea macrophylla* var. *thunbergii* (Hydrangeae Dulcis Folium) substantially inhibited the degranulations by antigen and calcium ionophore A23187, and the releases of TNF-alpha and IL-4 by antigen in RBL-2H3 cells. Phyllodulcin and hydrangenol also showed significant inhibition for the antigen-induced degranulations, but their effects were weaker than those of thunberginols A, B, and F. These active compounds inhibited the degranulation processes both before and after increase in intracellular free Ca2+ levels.	Wang et al., 2006	3
Hydrastis canadensis	Ethnoveterinary use -skin problems, abscesses, dog bites, bleeding wounds, sprains, post-operative bleeding, deep wounds, abrasions Berberine inhibited activator protein 1 (AP-1), a key transcription factor in inflammation and	Anon, 2000	3

	carcinogenesis. Berberine has a significant inhibitory effect on lymphocyte transformation, and its anti-inflammatory action may be due to inhibition of DNA synthesis in activated lymphocytes. During platelet activation in response to tissue injury, berberine has a direct affect on several aspects of the inflammatory process. It exhibits dose-dependent inhibition of arachidonic acid release from cell membrane phospholipids, inhibition of thromboxane A2 from platelets, and inhibition of thrombus formation.		
Hypericum perforatum	Ethnoveterinary use - sprains, post-operative bleeding, deep wounds, abrasions, surgery scars, raccoon in coma The plant contains hypericin with anti-H5N1 and H9N2 activity. A proantocyanidin fraction from *H. perforatum* antagonised histamine and PG F2alpha-induced arterial contractions. Hypericin and pseudohypericine (naphthodianthrones) have activity against animal retroviruses.	Wang et al., 2006; Tunón et al., 1995; Sydiskis et al., 1991	3
Juglans nigra	Ethnoveterinary use - rheumatoid arthritis, joint pain Ethanolic and aqueous extracts from some plant species were evaluated for *in vivo* anti-inflammatory and antinociceptive activities; *Juglans regia* L. leaves, *Rubus hirtus* Walds. et Kit aerial parts and *Rubus sanctus* Schreber aerial parts and roots. All the plant extracts, except the aqueous extract of *Rubus hirtus*, had significant antinociceptive activity in varying degrees against p-benzoquinone-induced abdominal contractions in mice.	Erdemoglu et al., 2003; Papoutsi et al., 2007	3

	However, only the ethanolic extracts of *Juglans regia* leaves, exhibited potent anti-inflammatory activity against carrageenan-induced hind paw edema model in mice without inducing any gastric damage. The plants possess potent antinociceptive and anti-inflammatory activity.		
Lactuca muralis	Ethnoveterinary use - rheumatoid arthritis, joint pain *L. virosa* has analgesic, antitussive and sedative properties attributed to the presence of sesquiterpene lactones. A number of sesquiterpene lactones and their glycosides have been reported from other *Lactuca* species.	Kisiel and Zielińska, 2000	2
Larrea tridentata	Ethnoveterinary use - rheumatoid arthritis, joint pain In the carrageenan-induced rat paw edema model of anti-inflammatory activity, a dose of 400 mg/kg of *Larrea tridentata* methanol extract was active against the induced hind-paw edema. Relatively small intakes of *Larrea* tincture, or topical application of extracts in Ricinus oil, may be safe if properly prescribed. *Larrea* should be used with caution in persons with liver disease. *Larrea* capsules have been associated with potentially dangerous overdosing. Actinex is a topical drug used for actinic keratoses derived from *Larrea tridentata*. Chaparral contains the compound nordihydroguairetic acid, which is useful as an antibiotic in the skin and elsewhere, and also has potent antioxidant properties.	Meckes et al., 2004; Heron and Yarnell, 2001; Dattner, 2003; Culver et al., 2005	3
Lavandula officinalis	Ethnoveterinary use -wounds, sprains, post-operative	Hajhashemi et al., 2003	3

	bleeding, abrasions Extracts, fractions and essential oil of *Lavandula angustifolia* are reported to have CNS-depressant, anti-convulsive, sedative and anti-bacterial effects.		
Lobelia inflata	Ethnoveterinary use - rheumatoid arthritis, joint pain Effects of beta-amyrin palmitate isolated from the leaves of *Lobelia inflata* were studied on the central nervous system of mice and were compared with those of antidepressant drugs, mianserin and imipramine. Beta-amyrin palmitate has some similar properties to mianserin and might possess sedative activity. *Lobelia inflata* contains linoleic acid which has a pro-inflammatory effect that may speed wound healing.	Subarnas et al., 1993; Philipov et al., 1998; Ma and Wink, 2008; Duke, 2008, Pereira et al., 2008	3
Mahonia aquifolium	Ethnoveterinary use -wounds, sprains, post-operative bleeding, abrasions Berberine can be used to treat ocular C.*trachomatis*. *Berberis vulgaris* and other *Berberis* species contain several alkaloids in their roots: jatrorrdizine, berberine, berberrubine, berbamine, bervulcine, palmatine, columbamine, and oxyacanthine, and also contain chelidonic, citric, malic, and tartaric acids. Berberine, berbamine and palmatine are the main antinociceptive, antipyretic and antiinflammatory compounds in the roots of *Berberis* species.	Vermani and Garg, 2002; Di et al., 2003; Küpeli et al., 2002	3
Medicago sativa	Ethnoveterinary use - rheumatoid arthritis, joint pain, dietary supplement for articular cartilage injury, partial tear of cruciate ligament, raccoon in coma *In vitro* experiments showed	Zhao et al., 1993	3

	that 250-500 micrograms/ml-1 of the polysaccharides isolated from *Medicago sativa* L., had immunopotentiating effects. The abilities of PWM-induced antibody production were elevated 51% and 78%, respectively.		
Melaleuca alternifolia	Ethnoveterinary use -wounds, sprains, post-operative bleeding, abrasions Tea tree oil was used as an adjunctive therapy in treating osteomyelitis and infected chronic wounds in case studies and small clinical trials.	Caldefie-Chezet et al., 2006; Halcon and Milkus, 2004	3
Origanum vulgare	Ethnoveterinary use -wounds, sprains, post-operative bleeding, abrasions *Origanum* x *majoricum* and *Origanum vulgare* ssp. *Hirtum* have higher phenolic contents compared to other culinary herbs. Rosmarinic acid is the predominant phenolic compound in *Salvia officinalis*, *Thymus vulgaris* and *Origanum* x *majoricum*.	Zheng and Wang, 2001	2
Plantago major	Ethnoveterinary use -snake bite, wounds, sprains, post-operative bleeding, abscesses; External treatment and anxiety associated with swollen anal gland Plantain seeds are said to stimulate macrophage activity (interferon inducers) and stimulate immunological systems and may improve endocrine dysfunction. Hot water extracts of *Plantago major* showed dual effects of immunodulatory activity, enhancing lymphocyte proliferation and secretion of interferon-gamma at low concentrations (< 50 microg/ml), but inhibiting this effect at high concentrations (> 50 microg/ml).	Kaji et al., 2004; Chiang et al., 2003; Hausmann et al., 2007	3

Prunella vulgaris	Ethnoveterinary use -wounds, sprains, post-operative bleeding, abrasions SKI 306X is a purified extract (containing *Clematis mandshurica*, *Trichosanthes kirilowii* and *Prunella vulgaris*). A double-blind, controlled study was performed to evaluate the efficacy and safety of SKI 306X with placebo in 96 patients with classical osteoarthritis of the knee. Patients were randomized to four treatment groups: placebo, 200 mg, 400 mg and 600 mg of SKI 306X t.i.d.. Clinical efficacy and safety were evaluated for 4 weeks continuous treatment. This study demonstrated that SKI 306X provided clinical efficacy in patients with osteoarthritis.	Jung et al., 2001	4
Rosa gymnocarpa	Ethnoveterinary use -gum inflammation from broken tooth *Rosa hybrida* flower has antioxidant activity. HDL-cholesterol significantly increased in the *Rosa hybrida* group of treated rats (daily intake of 0.2 g/kg body weight for 3 weeks). Anxiolytic-like properties were found in rose oil. *Rosa canina* has antibacterial activity against one pathogenic bacterial species. *Rosa rugosa* has hydrolysable tannins (in the leaves and petals), catechin derivatives (roots), flavonoids (leaves), 2-phenoxychromones (leaves), monoterpenes (floral parts, leaves), sesquiterpenes (leaves) and triterpenes (leaves and roots). *R. rugosa* accumulates heavy metals (Fe, Cu and Zn) in the leaves. Tocopherols and carotenes, antioxidants, are abundant in the leaves and fruits.	Choi and Hwang, 2005 ; de Almeida et al., 2004; Kumarasamy et al., 2002; Hashidoko, 1996	3
Rubus idaeus	Ethnoveterinary use -wounds, sprains, post-operative	Nam et al., 2006	3

	bleeding, abrasions This study was undertaken to ascertain the clinical merits of two natural antinociceptive anti-inflammatory triterpenoids. The triterpenoid glycoside niga-ichigoside F1 (NIF1) and its aglycone 23-hydroxytormentic acid (23-HTA), which were isolated from the unripe fruits of *Rubus coreanus*, showed an anti-rheumatic effect. They also had an anti-gastropathic effect attributed to free radical scavenging enzyme activities. These compounds did not show the adverse effects of synthetic anti-inflammatory drugs.		
Rumex crispus	Ethnoveterinary use -nettle stings, snake bites The antioxidant and antimicrobial activities of ether, ethanol, and hot water extracts of the leaves and seeds of *Rumex crispus* were studied. The antioxidant activities of the extracts increased with increasing dosages (50-150 microg). The water extracts of the leaves and seeds had the greatest antioxidant activities. More phenolic compounds were found in the ethanol extract of seeds. The ether extracts of both the leaves and seeds and the ethanol extract of leaves had antimicrobial activities on *S. aureus* and *B. subtilis*. None of the water extracts showed antimicrobial activity on the studied microorganisms.	Yildirim et al., 2001	3
Salix lucida	Ethnoveterinary use -articular cartilage injury Two moderate-quality trials utilizing *Salix alba* found moderate evidence for short-term improvements in pain and rescue medication for daily doses standardized to 120 mg or 240 mg salicin with an	Gagnier et al., 2006; Fiebich and Chrubasik, 2004	4

	additional trial demonstrating relative equivalence to 12.5 mg per day of rofecoxib.		
Salvia officinalis	Ethnoveterinary use -gum inflammation from broken tooth A Salvia-based extract demonstrated antibacterial activity against a variety of bacteria. Water-soluble polysaccharides from the leaves of *Plantago lanceolata*, and the aerial parts of *Salvia officinalis* showed immunomodulatory activities with the *in vitro* mitogenic and comitogenic rat thymocyte tests. The tested polysaccharides showed similar significant immunomodulatory properties with a particularly high adjuvans activity in the case of the *Salvia* polysaccharides.	Weckesser et al., 2007; Ebringerova et al., 2003; Juhás et al., 2008	3
Scutellaria lateriflora	Ethnoveterinary use -raccoon in coma The anti-inflammatory effect of Scutellaria Radix was studied and confirmed.	Chen et al., 2006; Hsieh et al., 2007	3
Smilax officinalis	Ethnoveterinary use - rheumatoid arthritis, joint pain The aqueous extract from Rhizoma Smilacis Glabrae (RSG) inhibited the primary inflammation of adjuvant arthritis (AA) in rats and may be advantageous to the long-term treatment of clinical rheumatoid arthritis. Four steroidal saponins were isolated from the BuOH extract of *Smilax china* L., along with 13 known compounds. All the compounds showed inhibitory effects on cyclooxygenase-2 enzyme (COX-2) activities at final concentration of 10^{-5}M, and one compound showed an inhibitory effect on production of TNFalpha (tumor necrosis factor alpha) in murine peritoneal macrophages at the	Jiang and Xu et al., 2003; Shao et al., 2007; Psotová et al., 2004	4

	same concentration.		
Stellaria media	Ethnoveterinary use -wounds, sprains, post-operative bleeding, abrasions Two cyclic peptides were isolated from the roots of *Stellaria dichotoma*, and they showed a moderate vasorelaxant effect on rat aorta.	Morita et al., 2005	3
Symphytum officinale	Ethnoveterinary use -abscesses, dog bites, bleeding wounds, sprains, post-operative bleeding, deep wounds, abrasions, articular cartilage injury, partial tear of cruciate ligament This randomised, double-blind, bicenter, placebo-controlled clinical trial investigated the effect of a daily application of 6g comfrey root extract (3 x 2 g) over a 3 week period on patients suffering from painful osteoarthritis of the knee (53 women and 67 men of an average age of 57.9 years). The results suggested that the comfrey root extract ointment is well suited for the treatment of osteoarthritis of the knee. Pain was reduced, mobility of the knee improved and quality of life increased.	Grube et al., 2007	4
Taraxacum officinale	Ethnoveterinary use – articular cartilage injury The most efficient inhibition of hydroxyl radical production was achieved with ethyl acetate and water extracts of dandelion flowers and aqueous dandelion stem extract. Pronounced inhibitory effects were also obtained using chloroform and ethyl acetate extracts of leaf and ether, or n-butanol extracts of roots.	Schütz et al., 2006	3
Ulmus fulva	Ethnoveterinary use -wounds, sprains, post-operative bleeding, abrasions, swollen anal gland	Cho et al., 2003; Son et al., 2004	3

	Ulmus parvifolia reduced lipid peroxidation more effectively as lipid peroxidation progressed. Excessive breakdown of extracellular matrix by metalloproteinases (MMPs) occurs in many pathological conditions. Consequently, methods for inhibiting MMP activity have therapeutic potential. The effect of G-120, a glycoprotein purified from *Ulmus davidiana* Nakai (UDN), on the activity and production of several MMPs was studied by evaluating its growth inhibitory effect on NIH 3T3 cells. G-120 strongly reduced the gelatinolytic and collagenase activities of MMP proteins, as well as expression of MMP-2 and MMP-9. It suppressed the DNA binding activity of NF-kappaB.		
Urtica dioica	Ethnoveterinary use- rheumatoid arthritis, joint pain, articular cartilage injury. *Urtica diocia* and willow bark extract are effective treatments for osteoarthritis. *Urtica diocia* decreases the production of TNF-alpha. *Urtica dioica* extract produced a dose-dependent inhibition of thrombin and ADP-induced aggregation. The calculated IC50 (half-maximal inhibition of thrombin and ADP-induced aggregation) was high for *Urtica dioica*. Polyphenolic compounds present in the extract may be involved in the treatment or prevention of platelet aggregation complications.	Setty and Sigal, 2005; Mekhfi et al., 2004; Chrubasik et al., 2007; Schulze-Tanzil et al., 2002	4
Usnea longissima	Ethnoveterinary use -External treatment and anxiety associated with swollen anal gland	Cansaran et al., 2006	3

	Six species of lichens: *Usnea florida, Usnea barbata, Usnea longissima, Usnea rigida, Usnea hirta* and *Usnea subflorida*, have antimicrobial activities against *E. coli*, *Enterococcus faecalis, Proteus mirabilis, S. aureus, Bacillus subtilis* and *Bacillus megaterium*. With increasing amount of usnic acid, the antimicrobial activity increased. Usnic acid contents of *Usnea* species varied between 0.22-6.49% of dry weight.		

TABLE 6. MOLECULAR TARGETS OF NATURAL PRODUCTS THAT EXHIBIT ANTI-ARTHRITIC POTENTIAL (ADAPTED AND EXPANDED FROM KHANNA ET AL., 2007)

Potential source	Plant compounds	Molecular targets found in testing some species	References
Harpagophytum procumbens, Lactuca sativa	Luteolin	NF-κB, COX-2, TNFalpha, IL-1beta	Kaszkin et al., 2004; Kisiel and Zielińska, 2000
Avena sativa, Capsicum frutescens, Allium sativum var. *sativum*	Quercetin	NF-κB, COX-2, TNF-alpha, 5-LOX, TNF-alpha, IL-1beta	Nie et al., 2006; Ji et al., 2003; Liu et al., 2004a; Vollmar, 2003
Symphytum officinale	Rosmarinic acid, allantoin, hydroxyl-cinamon acid derivatives	NF-κB, COX-2, TNF-alpha, AMs	Lohmann et al., 2000
Astragalus membranaceus	Polysaccharides, saponins	NF-κB, iNOS, COX-2, IL-6, IL-1beta	Barrett and Zwickey, 2006; Zhang et al., 2003
Hydrangea paniculata	Rutin	IL-1beta, NF-κB	Matsuda et al., 2008; Wang et al., 2006

Cimicifuga racemosa	25-acetylcimigenol xylopyranoside	IL-4, IL-5, TNF-alpha	Rhyu et al., 2006; Kim et al., 2004; Qui et al., 2007
Arctium lappa	Arctigenin	iNOS, NF-κB	Park et al., 2007
Fucus vesiculosus	Fucoidan	NF-κB	Ruperez et al., 2002; Kim and Joo, 2008.
Juglans nigra	Ellagic acid	TNF-alpha	Papoutsi et al., 2008
Larrea tridentata	Nordihydroguaiaretic acid	TNF-alpha	Culver et al., 2005
Lobelia laxiflora, Lobelia inflata	Lobeline, linoleic acid	PAF, IL-1beta	Ma and Wink, 2008
Salix lucida	Ethanolic Salix extract, lipophilic fraction	TNF-alpha, IL-1beta, IL-6,	Fiebich and Chrubasik, 2004
Smilax officinalis	Quercetin, kaempferol	IL-1, TNF-alpha	Jiang and Xu, 2003
Urtica dioica	13-Hydroxyoctadecatrienic acid	NF-κB, IL-1beta, MMP-9	Schulze-Tanzil et al., 2002

Key:

AM = adhesion molecule;

ICAM-1 = intercellular adhesion molecule

IL-1beta =Interleukin (IL)-1beta;

NF-κB = nuclear factor-kappa B

iNOS= inducible nitric oxide synthase;

MMP-9 = matrix metallopeptidase 9;   COX-2 = cycloxygenase-2

5-LOX = 5-lipoxygenase;

TNF-alpha = tumor necrosis factor

IL-6 = Interleukin 6

PAF = pro-inflammatory phospholipids

ETHNOVETERINARY REMEDIES USED IN BRITISH COLUMBIA, CANADA FOR MEGACOLON, URINARY, GASTROINTESTINAL, ENDOCRINOPATHIES AND HEPATIC DISEASES AND OTHER PROBLEMS IN DOGS AND CATS

Abstract

This chapter presents the plants reported to be used for gastrointestinal, urinary and other problems in dogs and cats. The plants used included ginger (*Zingiber officinale*), rosemary (*Rosmarinus officinalis*), fennel (*Foeniculum vulgare*), oregano (*Origanum majorana*), turmeric (*Curcuma longa*), gentian (*Gentiana lutea*), lemon balm (*Melissa officinalis*) and peppermint (*Mentha piperita*). Cushings/hyperadrenocorticism is treated with ginkgo leaf (*Ginkgo biloba*). Parsley piert (*Alchemilla arvensis*), Hydrangea (*Hydrangea arborescens*) and nettles (*Urtica dioica*) are used as kidney tonics.

Keywords: megacolon; benign hyperplasia, hepatic disease, pets; gastrointestinal problems; ethnoveterinary medicine; British Columbia

1. Introduction

This chapter focuses on the plants used for gastrointestinal, urinary and other problems in dogs and cats.

Interest in plant-based antimicrobial agents has arisen because of the interest in holistic medicine and organic farming, and because increasing on-farm use of antibiotics as growth promotors has reduced their effectiveness in hospitals. Some antibiotics also have side effects including allergic reactions and immune-suppression (Salamci et al., 2007). This makes the search for plant-based alternative antimicrobial agents more important.

Antimicrobial resistance was commonly found for penicillin G, lincomycin, tetracycline and trimethoprimsulphamethoxazole in both *Staphylococcus* species isolated from dogs in British Columbia (Hoekstra and Paulton, 2002). There was significant resistance to cloxacillin in *S. aureus* isolates. A total of 867 isolates of *S. aureus* and 1339 isolates of *S. intermedius* were obtained from the face, reproductive areas, urine, skin and throat isolates of dogs (specimens were obtained from a lab in British Columbia). *S. intermedius* isolates were most frequent. *Staphylococci* species are implicated in a wide variety of diseases in animals. British Columbia had a 4.1% Giardia prevalence in dogs in 1999 (Jacobs et al., 2001). Giardia and cryptosporidium infections are relatively common in pets, but most dogs and cats show few clinical signs. Giardiasis and Cryptosporidiosis in dogs and cats can result in small bowel diarrhoea (Thompson et al., 2007).

Commonly used culinary herbs have a long tradition of use for stomach ailments, one of the health problems being treated with ethnoveterinary remedies. In one study of culinary herbs coriander (*Coriandrum sativum*) and fenugreek (*Trigonella foenum-graecum*) had no bactericidal effect on *Helicobacter pylori* (one cause of gastroduodenal diseases), sage (*Salvia officinalis*) and cinnamon (*Cinnamomum verum*) had limited bactericidal activity while turmeric (*Curcuma longa*), followed by ginger (*Zingiber officinale*), oregano (*Origanum majorana*) and licorice (*Glycyrrhiza glabra*) killed the bacteria (O' Mahony et al., 2005). Extracts of turmeric inhibited the adhesion of *H. pylori* strains to the stomach sections (O' Mahony et al., 2005). Oregano in another study was active against one standard strain and 15 clinical isolates of *H. pylori* obtained from a Greek hospital (Stamatis et al., 2003).

Addison's disease and Cushing's syndrome were both successfully treated by a veterinarian in this study. Essential hypertension with raised blood pressure is increasing worldwide. 'Secondary' hypertension with a known cause is linked to adrenal corticosteroids (Hammer and Stewart, 2006). Hypoadrenocorticism (Addison's disease) in animals is caused by deficient secretion of endogenous glucocorticoid and mineralocorticoids (aldosterone), with many resulting clinical signs that may be mistaken for renal failure and various gastrointestinal disorders (Meeking, 2007; Greco, 2007). Naturally occurring primary hypoadrenocorticism in both cats and dogs is usually caused by immune-mediated destruction of the adrenal cortex. Secondary hypoadrenocorticism, in which the pituitary gland produces inadequate amounts of adrenocorticotrophic hormone (ACTH), can be caused by chronic steroid therapy or less commonly by tumors, trauma, or congenital defects of the pituitary gland. Inadequate secretion of corticosteroids in Addison's disease causes life threatening hypotension, whereas mineralocorticoid and glucocorticoid excess in primary hyperaldosteronism and Cushing's syndrome, respectively, result in high blood pressure (Hammer and Stewart, 2006). Cushing's disease results from glucocorticoid excess or is an indirect result of obesity (Meij et al., 1997). Dogs with the pituitary dependent Cushing's disease typically present with benign tumors but half of the tumors in adrenal Cushing's Syndrome are malignant (Zeugswetter et al., 2007).

2. Materials and methods

The methods used in this study are detailed in the introductory chapter.

3. Results

Table 7 documents the plants used in this study for kidney, liver and urinary problems in pets. Table 8 lists the treatments and dosages for kidney and liver problems in pets.

The treatments for gastrointestinal problems, constipation and megacolon in cats and dogs are presented in Table 9. Table 10 lists the treatment details for gastrointestinal problems, constipation and emesis in cats and dogs in British Columbia. Table 11 contains the non-experimental validation of plants used for megacolon, urinary, gastrointestinal, endocrinopathies and hepatic diseases and other problems in cats and dogs in British Columbia.

Treatments for benign hyperplasia and prostate support

Benign hyperplasia in dogs was successfully treated with 1 ml (¼ tsp) saw palmetto (*Serenoa repens*) fruit extract every day for four days (39 kg dog). The treatment was stopped for a few days and then restarted. A tea was made using 15 ml (1 tbsp) of berries in 0.46 L of water; 57 ml of the tea was put in the drinking water.

Plants used as a kidney tonic

A tonic for kidney complaints consisted of parsley piert (*Alchemilla arvensis*), root of hydrangea (*Hydrangea arborescens*), cornsilk (*Zea mays*) and nettles (*Urtica dioica*). Chopped hydrangea root (28 gm) was soaked overnight. The next day a decoction was made with 1 L of water (in a glass pot, simmered for 15 minutes). The decoction was supplemented with 29 gm each of parsley piert, cornsilk and nettles added in the last 5 minutes of simmering. A dog was given 57 ml of the strained decoction twice daily (per 11 to 14 kg patient bodyweight) for five days.

Treatments for a dog born with a tiny malformed kidney

This dog was given a tincture of nettles aerial parts (*Urtica dioica*) in 30% alcohol as a kidney tonic (10 drops twice daily per 23 kgs bodyweight for twelve months). This remedy and other homeopathic remedies (not presented) were claimed to have extended the life of the pet by ten months.

Treatments for Cushings/hyperadrenocorticism

Cushings/hyperadrenocorticism (an excess of cortisol produces the clinical signs excessive urination and thirst, panting) was diagnosed by a veterinarian in an 8-year-old patient (female Doberman X, 50 kgs). Capsules of ginkgo leaf (*Ginkgo biloba*) were administered by mouth (purchased human brand name product - 500 mg; 2/3 human dose used). After three weeks of treatment the veterinarian noticed less panting.

Treatments for urinary problems

A case study of incontinence linked to spaying; with blood in the urine. A veterinarian diagnosed the dog's condition. The pet was given a purchased uva-ursi (*Arctostaphylos uva-ursi*) tincture (20 drops twice a day). The pet was also given a 1:1 tincture of Oregon grape root (*Mahonia aquifolium*) twice a day to clear up bacteria in the urine. The 16 kg dog was given 10 drops/day for five days, to be repeated after five days, but the first five days was sufficient in this case.

Treatments for pets with liver problems

Pets with liver problems were given 60 – 80% alcoholic tincture of milk thistle seed (*Silybum marianum*) (30 drops twice a day). Alternatively the powdered seed was added to the pet's food, or seeds were ground and placed in capsules before administration. A tincture was made with 60 ml (¼ cup) seeds in 284 ml of vodka, brandy or rum (46 kg dog got 2.5 ml four times daily). This treatment was considered an early response for chronic liver problems.

Another dog (27 kg) was given 30 drops of each purchased herb tincture below per day (or 1 drop per 1 kg body weight per day by mouth). The tincture consisted of licorice root (*Glycyrrhiza glabra*), eleuthero root (*Eleutherococcus senticosus*), and wild yam root (*Dioscorea villosa*). An adrenal glandular supplement was given indefinitely as a supportive treatment. This dog was also given a purchased capsule that contained these ingredients: milk thistle seed (*Silybum marianum*), dandelion root (*Taraxacum officinale*), artichoke leaf (*Cynara scolymus*) and turmeric root (*Curcuma longa*).

Treatment for a dog with Addison's disease

A male Bouvier of 6 years old and weighing 34 kgs was diagnosed with Addison's disease (early hypoadrenocorticism) by a veterinarian. The symptoms were weakness, vomiting and diarrhoea at times of stress. Single tinctures of licorice root (*Glycyrrhiza glabra*), eleuthero root (*Eleutherococcus senticosus*) and wild yam root (*Dioscorea villosa*) were used. The dose was 30 drops tincture of each herb per day (ie: 1 drop per 1 kg body weight per day orally). Episodes of weakness, vomiting/diarrhoea were resolved after two weeks using the herbs. These episodes had been intermittent for the previous three years and did not recur in the six months after using the herbs. An adjunctive treatment was also used, consisting of a dried purchased product which is an adrenal glandular supplement (the pet had taken the product for three years prior to this research).

Treatment for urinary problems in dogs

For urinary problems a purchased product was used containing uva-ursi/bearberry (*Arctostaphylos uva-ursi*), bilberry (*Vaccinium myrtillus*) and juniper berries (*Juniperus communis*) (200 milligrams per 9 kgs body weight). This combination of herbs was not given during pregnancy or for serious kidney problems and was not given for longer than two weeks. For uva-ursi's effectiveness the pet's urine was made alkaline by including vegetables, fruit, fruit juices and potatoes in the pet's diet. Pets were given plenty of water to ease elimination and prevent renal calculi.

One dog breeder used a purchased kidney and blood pressure tea prepared by a local herbalist to treat her dogs. The ingredients are listed in Table 12. Other treatments and dosages for kidney and liver problems are given in Table 13.

Treatments for pets with gastrointestinal ailments

For gastrointestinal ailments (dyspepsia, gastritis, bloating, colic, flatulence, impaired digestion), a multi-ingredient decoction is made with 1 cinnamon stick (*Cinnamomum zeylandica*) steeped for 20 minutes in 500 ml of boiling water with 30 ml (2 tbsp) dried leaves of peppermint, then the leaves are removed and 5 ml (1 tsp) ginger powder (*Zingiber officinalis*), 30 ml (2 tbsp) dried leaves of peppermint, 5 ml (1 tsp) fennel seeds (*Foeniculum vulgare*), 5 ml (1 tsp) fenugreek seeds (*Trigonella foenum-graecum*), 1 ml (¼ tsp) ground cloves (*Eugenia caryophyllus*) are added and this is simmered on very low heat for an additional 30 minutes. Or a combination decoction is made with 1 ml (1 tsp) dried shredded gentian (*Gentiana lutea*) root, 1 ml (1 tsp) fennel seeds (*Foeniculum vulgare*) and 1 ml (1 tsp) ginger powder (*Zingiber officinalis*) in 750 ml of water. This is sweetened with honey. Another combined tea consists of 15 ml (1 tbsp) of chopped sage leaf (*Salvia officinalis*), 1 stick of cinnamon and 1 bay leaf (*Laurus nobilis*) added to 500 ml of boiling water.

Treatments for chronic constipation

A case of megacolon was diagnosed and treated by a veterinarian. The patient was a 14 year old male domestic long-haired cat, 12.3 kgs, with constipation. Megacolon is an abnormal widening of the colon. The treatment used was intended to deal with the symptoms and not as a long-term cure.

A tincture was made with 4 parts cascara bark (*Rhamnus purshiana*), 1 part ginger root (*Zingiber officinalis*) and 2 parts diglycerised licorice root (*Glycyrrhiza glabra*). The dose used was 0.1 ml per 2.3 kgs twice for 1 day (0.5 ml every 12 hours for this cat). The cat was also given capsules of slippery elm bark powder bark (*Ulmus fulva*) and marshmallow root (*Althaea officinalis*) (1/8th a human dose). The cat did not get constipated while on these herbs, and became constipated again when they were stopped. An adjunctive treatment for the cat consisted of vitamin C (which produces diarrhoea in cats) (NB: the cat was also diabetic and obese). Four parts cascara bark (a relatively large dose) was specific to this case and is not a recommendation for other pets.

A tea for another cat with constipation was made with 15 ml (1 tbsp) dried bark of cascara (*Frangula purshiana*), 15 ml (1 tbsp) fresh stem of rhubarb (*Rheum palmatum*), 15 ml (1 tbsp) fresh root of yellow dock (*Rumex crispus*), 2 ml (½ tsp) psyllium seeds (*Plantago psyllium*) and 0.45 litres of chicken broth (5 ml (1 tsp) three times a day for a 5 kg cat). The dose was increased as needed to induce a bowel movement. Canned food was supplemented with 25 mg magnesium and 2 ml (½ tsp) fish oil or flaxseed oil (*Linum usitatissium*).

4. Discussion

The non-experimental validation of the plants, presented in Table 5 indicates that the majority of these ethnoveterinary uses are supported by the literature. Some of the plants used are discussed in more detail below.

Benign hyperplasia in dogs was one condition treated with ethnoveterinary remedies in British Columbia. Steenkamp et al. (2006) reported that prostatitis (inflammation of the prostate, acute bacterial prostatitis, chronic bacterial prostatitis and chronic non-bacterial prostatitis), and benign prostatic hyperplasia (BPH) (enlargement of the prostate due to non-cancerous growth within the gland), are common prostate disorders (in humans). Chronic non-bacterial prostatitis is common and is usually caused by fungi, mycoplasmas or viruses. Acute bacterial prostatitis is caused by a urinary tract infection, typically *Escherichia coli*, which has spread to the prostate, and chronic bacterial prostatitis is often the result of partial blockage of the male urinary tract, with the resulting proliferation of bacteria. BPH has two phases, one with no clinical signs and the second demonstrated as disorders of urination resulting from urinary tract obstruction by an enlarged prostate (Steenkamp et al., 2006). BPH is often associated with a hormone-induced chronic inflammation that results from the infiltration of inflammatory cells (and prostaglandins, leukotrienes and growth factors) into the prostate. Agents such as a lipidosterolic extract of saw palmetto (*Serenoa repens*) are equivalent to tamsulosin in the treatment of BPH. In a comparison with finasteride, *Serenoa repens* extract had little effect on androgendependent parameters, but both treatments relieved the symptoms of BPH in two thirds of human patients (Hutchison et al., 2007).

Mahady et al. (2005) studied the *in vitro* susceptibility of 15 *Helicobacter pylori* strains to herbs with a history of use for gastrointestinal disorders. Methanol extracts of ginger rhizome/root (*Zingiber officinale*) and rosemary leaf (*Rosmarinus officinalis*) had an MIC of 25 microg/mL. Methanol extracts of herbs with a MIC of 50 microg/mL included fennel seed (*Foeniculum vulgare*), *Origanum majorana* (aerial parts) and a (1:1) combination of tumeric root (*Curcuma longa*) and ginger rhizome (*Zingiber officinale*). Herbs with a MIC of 100 microg/mL included gentian roots (*Gentiana lutea*), lemon balm leaves (*Melissa officinalis*) and peppermint leaves (*Mentha piperita*). All of these plants were used in the ethnoveterinary research in BC for stomach problems (see Lans et al., 2007 for the herbal remedies based on these plants that have been already published).

Watt et al. (2007) used two whole cell *Escherichia coli* luminescent biosensors to determine the antibacterial actions of 16 herbal tinctures (derived from culinary herbs and spices). They found that *Althaea officinalis* affected microbial metabolism and was 2–3-fold more effective than controls. This means the herb is more than just a demulcent. *Rosmarinus officinalis, Foeniculum vulgare, Trigonella foenum-graecum, Salvia triloba, Salvia officinalis*, and *Thymus vulgaris* were active against both strains. *Zingiber officinale* had weak activity against one of the strains. *Glycyrrhiza glabra* had a 4–5-fold greater antibacterial activity than controls. This herb is used successfully in the treatment of gastric ulcers.

Helicobacter pylori are Gram negative bacteria associated with gastric ulcers (Fukai et al., 2002). Glabridin and glabrene (from *Glycyrrhiza glabra*), licochalcone A (*Glycyrrhiza inflata*), licoricidin and licoisoflavone B (*Glycyrrhiza uralensis*) can inhibit the growth of *Helicobacter pylori in vitro*. These flavonoids also showed anti-*H. pylori* activity against a clarithromycin (CLAR) and amoxicillin (AMOX)-resistant strain. The activity of *T. foenum-graecum* on gastric ulcers might be explained by its phenolic content (Watt et al., 2007; Randhir and Shetty, 2007; Khayyal et al., 2001).

Acute hepatotoxicity induces inflammation, necrosis and oxidative stress of hepatocytes. Scientists currently believe that hepatocellular injury is not caused by the damaging agent itself but by the inflammatory cells that have been attacked by the stressed hepatocytes (Muriel and Rivera-Espinoza, 2007). Globe artichoke (*Cynara scolymus*) is traditionally used to treat human hepato-biliary diseases (Speroni et al., 2003). This activity is attributed to the antioxidative activity of artichoke extracts or to active compounds such as flavones, flavanones, flavonols, coumarins and phenolic acids. Artichoke's choleretic activity is attributed to mono- and di-caffeoylquinic acids. Chlorogenic acid from artichoke did not show liver protective activity (Speroni et al., 2003). Goñi et al. (2005) claims that artichoke's beneficial effects on intestinal health are actually due to artichoke's indigestible fraction which may enhance the activity of beneficial species in the colonic microbiota.

Eleutherococcus root (*Eleutherococcus senticosus*), an adaptogen with immunomodulative activity attributed to polysaccharides, is widely used to treat hepatitis (Park et al., 2004). A hot water extract of *E. senticosus* reduced the levels of aspartate transaminase and alanine transaminase in serum and improved histological changes of liver in induced liver injury in rats. *E. senticosus* inhibits tumour necrosis factor and iplatelet aggregation. Hot water extracts are also reported to inhibit mast cell-mediated anaphylaxis, induce apoptosis in human stomach cancer KATO III cells, and protect against gastric ulcers in stressed rats. Park et al. (2004) concluded that water-soluble polysaccharides of *E. senticosus* stems have protective effects against induced fulminant hepatic failure in mice. This finding justifies their ethnoveterinary use for liver problems in dogs.

Serenoa serrulata were used in the treatment of both BPH and prostatitis. It has hydroxyl scavenging activity which is reported to suppress upregulation of cyclooxygenase (COX) and subsequently reduce inflammation. Over-expression of COX-2 and a decrease in prostaglandin E-1 synthesis takes place in patients with BPH and prostatitis and the aqueous extracts of *Serenoa serrulata* showed a COX-2 inhibitory effect (Steenkamp et al., 2006). The Gram negative bacteria *Escherichia coli*, is a pathogen in cases of BPH and prostatitis, but the crude extract of *Serenoa serrulata* had no effect against it. A large study with men found that *Serenoa repens* was not better than placebo in the treatment of BPH (Bent et al., 2006). The study was criticized for the type of supplement used and because it included patients with moderate-to-severe BPH symptoms, when *Serenoa serrulata* is recommended for mild-to-moderate symptoms (ABC, 2006).

Quercetin and its sugar conjugates are commonly found bioflavonoids (Chander et al., 2005). Previous studies have shown that the polyphenol curcumin from turmeric (*Curcuma longa*) can decrease the degree of inflammation associated with experimental colitis (Camacho-Barquero et al., 2007). Conflicting results have been found in studies dealing with the benefits of curcumin in different nephrotoxic models of kidney injury. ADR-induced kidney injury in rats was prevented by treatment with curcumin (Venkatesan et al., 2000). Curcumin prevented renal lesions in streptozotocin diabetic rats and reduces ischaemic renal injury. In cyclosporin-induced acute renal failure, curcumin suspended in low concentration of 5, 10 and 15 mg/kg for 21 days, attenuated oxidative stress as well as BUN and serum creatinine (Vlahović et al., 2007). In a randomized, placebo-controlled trial, a combination of 480 mg curcumin and 20 mg quercetin was administered orally in capsule form to cadaveric kidney transplant recipients for 1 month, starting immediately after transplantation. The trial's 43 subjects were randomly assigned to placebo (control), low dose (one capsule + one placebo), or high dose (two capsule) regimens. The investigators observed better early graft function in treated patients than in controls (71% [lowdose] versus 93% [high-dose] versus 43% [controls]) and the high-dose regimen lowered the incidence of acute graft rejection at 6 months post-transplantation (0% versus 14.3%) (Goel et al. 2007).

Herbal remedies based on goldenrod (*Solidago virgaurea*) have been used for centuries to treat urinary tract diseases, and it was included in a multi-plant kidney and blood pressure tea in our research. Melzig (2004) claims that herbal preparations with a complex action spectrum (anti-inflammatory, antimicrobial, diuretic, antispasmodic, analgesic) should be used for treatment of infections and inflammations, to prevent formation of kidney stones and to help remove urinary gravel. Melzig (2004) concludes that goldenrod therapy is safe, is reasonably priced and does not show drug-related side-effects in humans.

5. Conclusion

Medicinal and culinary plants have long been used for gastrointestinal disorders, and the plants used for pets mirror those used for humans. The plants used for urinary and kidney problems showed efficacy in the non-experimental validation process. Quercetin, an extract from ginkgo leaves (*Ginkgo biloba*) supports kidney function due to its antioxidant and free radicals scavenging properties (Vlahović et al., 2007; Chandler et al., 2005). Curcumin has multiple therapeutic activities that are beneficial for kidney function (Venkatesan et al., 2000). Curcumin is safe even when consumed at a daily dose of 12 g for 3 months (Goel et al., 2007).

Conventional medicine has few therapeutic agents for treating hepato-biliary diseases (Aktay et al., 2000; Muriel and Rivera-Espinoza, 2007); holistic and other practitioners rely on milk thistle (*Silybum marianum*) and globe artichoke (*Cynara scolymus*), two of the plants used in this research. *Silybum marianum* is the most commonly used plant-based treatment for chronic or acute liver disease which has no major side-effects. Clinical trials have shown that silymarin is effective in treating various forms of liver disease, including cirrhosis, hepatitis, necroses, and liver damage induced by drug and alcohol abuse (Lee et al., 2006), as well as liver damage brought about from mushroom poisoning. It has several activities (antioxidative, antilipid peroxidative, membrane stabilizing, immunomodulatory and liver regeneration) (Muriel and Rivera-Espinoza, 2007). Silymarin is also useful for drug-induced nephrotoxicity in dogs that produces oxidative stress and leads to renal failure (Varzi et al., 2007).

Alternative treatments for Addison's disease and Cushing's syndrome are also useful. The literature review revealed that standardized *Ginkgo biloba* extract and its purified components, gingkolide A or ginkgolide B, can regulate glucocorticoid levels by controlling adrenal PBR expression at the transcriptional level. The extract and its purified component ginkgolide B decrease stress-induced elevations of serum corticosterone without affecting physiological basal levels and the extract contains an additional component that can regulate ACTH secretion (Amri et al., 2004).

The ethnoveterinary uses are supported in the literature. In our study *Althaea officinalis* achieved level 2 validity but all the other plants achieved a level 3 validity. The herbs documented here for use on dogs and cats have few safety issues, are easily obtained commercially and affordable to use in animal health.

References

Acuña UM, Atha DE, Ma J, Nee MH, Kennelly EJ. 2002. Antioxidant capacities of ten edible North American plants. Phytother Res. 16:63-5.

Ajith, T.A., Nivitha, V., Usha, S. 2007. *Zingiber officinale* Roscoe alone and in combination with alpha-tocopherol protect the kidney against cisplatin-induced acute renal failure. Food Chem Toxicol. 45:921-7.

Aktay, G., Deliorman, D., Ergun, E., Ergun, F., Yeşilada, E., Çevik, C., 2000. Hepatoprotective effects of Turkish folk remedies on experimental liver injury. J Ethnopharmacol. 73,121-9.

Ali, B.H., Blunden, G., Tanira, M.O., Nemmar, A., 2008. Some phytochemical, pharmacological and toxicological properties of ginger (*Zingiber officinale* Roscoe): A review of recent research. Food Chem Toxicol. 46(2),409-20.

Al-Mofleh, I.A., Alhaider, A.A., Mossa, J.S., Al-Sohaibani, M.O., Rafatullah S., Qureshi S., 2006. Protection of gastric mucosal damage by *Coriandrum sativum* L. pretreatment in Wistar albino rats. Environmental Toxicology and Pharmacology 22, 64-69.

Alcaraz MJ, Jiménez MJ. 1988. Protective effects of hypolaetin-8-glucoside on the rat gastric mucosa. Prog Clin Biol Res. 280:183-6.

Añón MT, Ubeda A, Alcaraz MJ. 1992. Protective effects of phenolic compounds on CCl4-induced toxicity in isolated rat hepatocytes. Z Naturforsch [C]. 47(3-4):275-9.

American Botanical Council, 2006. New clinical trial on saw palmetto inconsistent with positive results in previous studies. http://www.herbalgram.org/default.asp?c=sawpalmBPH

Amin, A., Hamza, A.A. 2005. Hepatoprotective effects of *Hibiscus*, *Rosmarinus* and *Salvia* on azathioprine-induced toxicity in rats. Life Sci. 77:266-78.

Amri, H., Drieu, K., Papadopoulos, V. 2003. Transcriptional suppression of the adrenal cortical peripheral-type benzodiazepine receptor gene and inhibition of steroid synthesis by ginkgolide B. Biochem Pharmacol. 65:717-29.

Amri, H., Li, W., Drieu, K., Papadopoulos, V. 2004. Identification of the adrenocorticotropin and ginkgolide B-regulated 90-kilodalton protein (p90) in adrenocortical cells as a serotransferrin precursor protein homolog (adrenotransferrin). Endocrinology 145:1802-9.

Anon, 2000. Berberine monograph. Alternative Medicine Review 5:175 – 177.

Anon, 2006. Monograph. *Eleutherococcus senticosus*. Altern Med Rev. 11:151-5.

Aydin, S., Beis, R., Ozturk, Y., Baser, K.H., Baser, C., 1998. Nepetalactone: A new opioid analgesic from *Nepeta caesarea* Boiss. J Pharm Pharmacol. 50,813-7.

Ball, K.R., Kowdley, K.V. 2005. A review of *Silybum marianum* (milk thistle) as a treatment for alcoholic liver disease. J Clin Gastroenterol. 39:520-8.

Bao, L., Yao, X.S., Tsi, D., Yau, C.C., Chia, C.S., Nagai, H., Kurihara, H. 2008. Protective effects of bilberry (*Vaccinium myrtillus* L.) extract on KBrO3-induced kidney damage in mice. J Agric Food Chem. 56:420-5.

Beaux, D., Fleurentin, J., Mortier, F. 1999. Effect of extracts of *Orthosiphon stamineus* Benth, *Hieracium pilosella* L., *Sambucus nigra* L. and *Arctostaphylos uva-ursi* (L.) Spreng. in rats. Phytother Res. 13(3):222-5.

Benghuzzi, H., Tucci, M., Eckie, R., Hughes, J. 2003. The effects of sustained delivery of diosgenin on the adrenal gland of female rats. Biomed Sci Instrum. 39:335-40.

Bent, S., Kane, C., Shinohara, K., Neuhaus, J., Hudes, E.S., Goldberg, H., Avins, A.L. 2006. Saw palmetto for benign prostatic hyperplasia. N Engl J Med. 354:557-66.

Blumenthal, M. 2000. Interactions Between Herbs and Conventional Drugs: Introductory Considerations. In: Herbs—everyday reference for health professionals. Ottawa: Canadian Pharmacists Association and Canadian Medical Association. pp. 9-20.

Bock, S., 2000. Integrative medical treatment of inflammatory bowel disease. Int J Integr Med. 2,21-29.

Boerth, J., Strong, K.M. 2002. The clinical utility of milk thistle (*Silybum marianum*) in cirrhosis of the liver. J Herb Pharmacother. 2,11-7.

Bonjar, G.H., 2004. Inhibition of Clotrimazole-resistant *Candida albicans* by plants used in Iranian folkloric medicine. Fitoterapia 75,74-6.

Bouidida el H., Alaoui. K., Cherrah, Y., Fkih-Tetouani, S., Idrissi, A.I., 2006. Acute toxicity and analgesic activity of the global extracts of *Nepeta atlantica* Ball and *Nepeta tuberosa* L. ssp. reticulata (Desf.) Maire. Therapie. 61,447-52. Article in French.

Bub, S., Brinckmann, J., Cicconetti, G., Valentine, B. 2006. Efficacy of an herbal dietary supplement (Smooth Move) in the management of constipation in nursing home residents: A randomized, double-blind, placebo-controlled study. J Am Med Dir Assoc. 7(9):556-61.

Bucar, F., Schneider, I., Ögmundsdóttir, H., Ingólfsdóttir, K., 2004. Anti-proliferative lichen compounds with inhibitory activity on 12(S)-HETE production in human platelets. Phytomedicine 11, 602-6.

Calixto, J.B., Beirith, A., Ferreira, J., Santos, A.R., Filho, V.C., Yunes, R.A., 2000. Naturally occurring antinociceptive substances from plants. Phytother Res. 14,401-18.

Camacho-Barquero, L., Villegas, I. Sánchez-Calvo, J.M., Talero, E., Sánchez-Fidalgo, S., Motilva, M., Alarcón de la Lastra, C. 2007. Curcumin, a *Curcuma longa* constituent, acts on MAPK p38 pathway modulating COX-2 and iNOS expression in chronic experimental colitis. Int Immunopharmacol 7:333-42.

Celik, I., Tuluce, Y., 2007. Elevation protective role of *Camellia sinensis* and *Urtica dioica* infusion against trichloroacetic acid-exposed in rats. Phytother Res. 21,1039-44.

Cervenka, L., Peskova, I., Foltynova, E., Pejchalova, M., Brozkova, I., Vytrasova, J., 2006. Inhibitory effects of some spice and herb extracts against *Arcobacter butzleri*, *A. cryaerophilus*, and *A. skirrowii*. Curr Microbiol. 53,435-9.

Chaieb, K., Hajlaoui, H., Zmantar, T., Kahla-Nakbi, A.B., Rouabhia, M., Mahdouani, K., Bakhrouf, A., 2007. The chemical composition and biological activity of clove essential oil, *Eugenia caryophyllata* (*Syzigium aromaticum* L. Myrtaceae): A short review. Phytother Res. 21,501-6.

Chander, V., Singh, D., Chopra, K. 2005. Reversal of experimental myoglobinuric acute renal failure in rats by quercetin, a bioflavonoid. Pharmacology. 73:49-56.

Chang, H.F., Lin, Y.H., Chu, C.C., Wu, S.J., Tsai, Y.H., Chao, J.C. 2007. Protective Effects of *Ginkgo biloba*, *Panax ginseng*, and *Schizandra chinensis* extract on liver injury in rats. Am. J. Chin. Med. 35: 995-1009.

Chen, H., Wang, C., Chang, C.T., Wang, T. 2003. Effects of Taiwanese yam (*Dioscorea japonica* Thunb var. *pseudojaponica* Yamamoto) on upper gut function and lipid metabolism in Balb/c mice. Nutrition 19:646-51.

Chethankumar M, Salimath PV, Sambaiah K. 2002. Butyric acid modulates activities of intestinal and renal disaccharidases in experimentally induced diabetic rats. Nahrung. 46(5):345-8.

Chithra, V., Leelamma, S., 2000. *Coriandrum sativum*--effect on lipid metabolism in 1,2-dimethyl hydrazine induced colon cancer. J Ethnopharmacol. 71. 457-63.

Cho, M.K., Jang, Y.P., Kim, Y.C., Kim, S.G. 2004. Arctigenin, a phenylpropanoid dibenzylbutyrolactone lignan, inhibits MAP kinases and AP-1 activation via potent MKK inhibition: the role in TNF-alpha inhibition. International Journal of Immunopharmacology 4: 1419-29.

Chun, S-S., Vattem, D.A., Lin, Y-T. and Shetty, K., 2005. Phenolic antioxidants from clonal oregano (*Origanum vulgare*) with antimicrobial activity against *Helicobacter pylori*. Process Biochemistry 40, 809-816.

Cowan, M.M., 1999. Plant products as antimicrobial agents. Clinical Microbiology Reveiws 12, 564–582.

Craig, W.J., 1999. Health-promoting properties of common herbs. Am J Clin Nutr. 70 (suppl), 491S–9S.

De Smet, P.A.G.M, D'Arcy, P.F., 1996. Drug interactions with herbal and other non-orthodox remedies. In: D'Arcy, P.F., McElnay, J.C., Welling, P.G., (editors) *Mechanisms of Drug Interactions*. New York: Springer-Verlag. pp. 327-52.

Desplaces, A., Choppin, J., Vogel, G., Trost, W. 1975. The effects of silymarin on experimental phalloidine poisoning. Arzneimittelforschung 25:89-96.

Dhiman, R.K., Chawla, Y.K., 2005. Herbal medicines for liver diseases. Dig Dis Sci. 50,1807-12.

Do Monte, F.H., dos Santos, J.G. Jr, Russi, M., Lanziotti, V.M., Leal, L.K., Cunha, G.M. 2004. Antinociceptive and anti-inflammatory properties of the hydroalcoholic extract of stems from *Equisetum arvense* L. in mice. Pharmacological Research (Lon) 49 (3): 239-43.

Dreikorn, K. 2002. The role of phytotherapy in treating lower urinary tract symptoms and benign prostatic hyperplasia. World J Urol. 19:426-35.

Duke JA. 1990. Promising phytomedicinals. In: J. Janick and J.E. Simon (eds.), Advances in new crops. Timber Press, Portland, OR. p. 491-498.

Duke, J. A., 2008. Phytochemical and Ethnobotanical Databases. USDA-ARS-NGRL, Beltsville Agricultural Research Center, Beltsville, Maryland, USA.

El-Ashmawy, I.M., Ashry, K.M., El-Nahas, A.F., Salama, O.M. 2006. Protection by turmeric and myrrh against liver oxidative damage and genotoxicity induced by lead acetate in mice. Basic Clin Pharmacol Toxicol. 98:32-7.

Farombi, E.O., Shrotriya, S., Na, H.K., Kim, S.H., Surh, Y.J. 2007. Curcumin attenuates dimethylnitrosamine-induced liver injury in rats through Nrf2-mediated induction of heme oxygenase-1. Food Chem Toxicol. 46(4):1279-87.

Ferrándiz ML, Alcaraz MJ. 1991. Anti-inflammatory activity and inhibition of arachidonic acid metabolism by flavonoids. Agents Actions. 32(3-4):283-8.

Filburn, C.R., Kettenacker, R., Griffin, D.W. 2007. Bioavailability of a silybin-phosphatidylcholine complex in dogs. J Vet Pharmacol Ther. 30:132-8.

Fukai, T., Marumo, A., Kaitou, K., Kanda, T., Terada, S., Nomura, T., 2002. Anti-*Helicobacter pylori* flavonoids from licorice extract. Life Sci. 71, 1449-63.

Galisteo, M., Suárez, A., Montilla, M.P, Fernandez, M.I., Gil, A., Navarro, M.C. 2006. Protective effects of *Rosmarinus tomentosus* ethanol extract on thioacetamide-induced liver cirrhosis in rats. Phytomedicine 13:101-8.

Geraghty, M., 2000. Herbal supplements for renal patients: What do we know? March 2000 Nephrology News & Issues.

Getie, M., Gebre-Mariam, T., Rietz, R., Hohne, C., Huschka, C., Schmidtke, M., Abate, A., Neubert, R.H. 2003. Evaluation of the anti-microbial and anti-inflammatory activities of the medicinal plants *Dodonaea viscosa*, *Rumex nervosus* and *Rumex abyssinicus*. Fitoterapia. 74,139-43.

Ghayur, M.N., Gilani, A.H., Khan, A., Amor, E.C., Villasenor, I.M., Choudhary, M.I., 2006. Presence of calcium antagonist activity explains the use of *Syzygium samarangense* in diarrhoea. Phytother Res. 20,49-52.

Goel, A., Kunnumakkara, A.B., Aggarwal, B.B. 2007. Curcumin as "Curecumin": From kitchen to clinic. Biochem Pharmacol. 75(4):787-809

Goñi, I. Jiménez-Escrig, A. Gudiel, M. Saura-Calixto, F. 2005. Artichoke (L) modifies bacterial enzymatic activities and antioxidant status in rat cecum. Nutrition Research 25: 607-615 I.

Graefe, E.U., Veit, M. 1999. Urinary metabolites of flavonoids and hydroxycinnamic acids in humans after application of a crude extract from *Equisetum arvense*. Phytomedicine 6: 239 - 46.

Greco, D.S. 2007. Hypoadrenocorticism in small animals. Clin Tech Small Anim Pract. 22:32-5.

Gudej J. 1991. Flavonoids, Phenolic Acids and Coumarins from the Roots of *Althaea officinalis*. Planta Med. 57(3):284-5.

Gupta, V.K., Fatima, A., Faridi, U., Negi, A.S., Shanker, K., Kumar, J.K., Rahuja, N., Luqman, S., Sisodia, B.S., Saikia, D., Darokar, M.P., Khanuja, S.P., 2008. Antimicrobial potential of *Glycyrrhiza glabra* roots. J Ethnopharmacol. 116(2):377-80.

Habtemariam, S. 1998. Extract of corn silk (stigma of *Zea mays*) inhibits the tumour necrosis factor-α- and bacterial lipopolysaccharide-induced cell adhesion and ICAM-1 expression. Planta Medica 64 (4): 314 - 318.

Habtemariam, S. 2001. Antiinflammatory activity of the antirheumatic herbal drug, gravel root (*Eupatorium purpureum*): further biological activities and constituents. Phytother Res 15(8):687-90.

Hajhashemi V, Abbasi N. 2008. Hypolipidemic activity of *Anethum graveolens* in rats. Phytother Res. 22(3):372-5.

Hammer, F., Stewart, P.M. 2006. Cortisol metabolism in hypertension. Best Pract Res Clin Endocrinol Metab. 20:337-53.

Hersch-Martinez, P., Leanos-Miranda, B.E., Solorzano-Santos, F., 2005. Antibacterial effects of commercial essential oils over locally prevalent pathogenic strains in Mexico. Fitoterapia 76,453-7.

Hoekstra, K.A., Paulton, R.J., 2002. Clinical prevalence and antimicrobial susceptibility of *Staphylococcus aureus* and *Staph. intermedius* in dogs. J Appl Microbiol. 93,406-13.

Hoffman, D. 2003. Medical Herbalism – The science and practice of herbal medicine. Healing Arts Press: Canada.

Holetz, F.B., Pessini, G.L., Sanches, N.R., Cortez, D.A., Nakamura, C.V., Filho, B.P. 2002. Screening of some plants used in the Brazilian folk medicine for the treatment of infectious diseases. Memorias do Instituto Oswaldo Cruz 97(7): 1027-31.

Hosseinzadeh, H., Karimi, G.R., Ameri, M., 2002. Effects of *Anethum graveolens* L. seed extracts on experimental gastric irritation models in mice. BMC Pharmacol. 2,21.

Hsu, J.H., Wu, Y.C., Liu, I.M., Cheng, J.T. 2007. Dioscorea as the principal herb of Die-Huang-Wan, a widely used herbal mixture in China, for improvement of insulin resistance in fructose-rich chow-fed rats. J Ethnopharmacol. 112:577-84.

Hussein, G., Miyashiro, H., Nakamura, N., Hattori, M., Kakiuchi, N., Shimotohno, K., 2000. Inhibitory effects of Sudanese medicinal plant extracts on Hepatitis C Virus (HCV) protease. Phytotherapy Research 14, 510 – 516.

Hutchison, A., Farmer, R., Verhamme, K., Berges, R., Navarrete, R.V. 2007. The efficacy of drugs for the treatment of LUTS/BPH, a study in 6 European countries. Eur Urol. 51:207-15.

Ingólfsdóttir, K., Chung, G.A., Skúlason, V.G., Gissurarson, S.R., Vilhelmsdóttir, M., 1998. Antimycobacterial activity of lichen metabolites *in vitro*. Eur J Pharm Sci. 6,141-4.

Jacobs, S.R., Forrester, C.P., Yang, J., 2001. A survey of the prevalence of Giardia in dogs presented to Canadian veterinary practices. Can Vet J. 42, 45-6.

Janicsák, G., Veres, K., Kakasy, A.Z., Máthé, I., 2006. Study of the oleanolic and ursolic acid contents of some species of the Lamiaceae. Biochemical Systematics and Ecology 34, 392-396.

Jellinek, N., Maloney, M. 2005. Escharotic and other botanical agents for the treatment of skin cancer: A review. J Am Acad Dermatol 53: 487-95.

Jiang, W.X., Xue, B.Y. 2005. Hepatoprotective effects of *Gentiana scabra* on the acute liver injuries in mice. Zhongguo Zhong Yao Za Zhi. 30(14):1105-7. Article in Chinese.

Kang, D.G., Sohn, E.J., Moon, M.K., Lee, Y.M., Lee, H.S. 2005. *Rehmannia glutinose* ameliorates renal function in the ischemia/reperfusion-induced acute renal failure rats. Biol Pharm Bull. 28:1662-7.

Khayyal, M.T., el-Ghazaly, M.A., Kenawy, S.A., Seif-el-Nasr, M., Mahran, L.G., Kafafi, Y.A., Okpanyi, S.N., 2001. Antiulcerogenic effect of some gastrointestinally acting plant extracts and their combination. Arzneimittelforschung. 51, 545-53.

Kim, H.Y., Kang, M.H. 2005. Screening of Korean medicinal plants for lipase inhibitory activity. Phytother Res. 19:359-61.

Koch E. 2001. Extracts from fruits of saw palmetto (*Sabal serrulata*) and roots of stinging nettle (*Urtica dioica*): Viable alternatives in the medical treatment of benign prostatic hyperplasia and associated lower urinary tracts symptoms. Planta Med. 67:489-500.

Kreydiyyeh, S.I., Usta, J. 2002. Diuretic effect and mechanism of action of parsley. Journal of Ethnopharmacology 79: 353-7.

Langmead, L., Dawson, C., Hawkins, C., Banna, N., Loo, S., Rampton, D.S., 2002. Antioxidant effects of herbal therapies used by patients with inflammatory bowel disease: an *in vitro* study. Aliment Pharmacol Ther. 16,197-205.

Lans, C., Turner, N., Brauer, G., Lourenco, G., Georges, K. 2006. Ethnoveterinary medicines used for horses in Trinidad and in British Columbia, Canada. Journal of Ethnobology and Ethnomedicine 2:31.

Lans, C., Turner, N., Khan, T., Brauer, G., 2007. Ethnoveterinary medicines used to treat endoparasites and stomach problems in pigs and pets in British Columbia, Canada. Vet. Parasitol 148, 325–340.

Lee, D.Y.W., Zhang, X., Ji, X.S. 2006. Preparation of tritium-labeled Silybin-a protectant for common liver diseases. J Label Compd Radiopharm 49:1125–1130.

Lieber, C.S., Leo, M.A., Cao, Q., Ren, C., DeCarli, LM. 2003. Silymarin retards the progression of alcohol-induced hepatic fibrosis in baboons. J Clin Gastroenterol. 37:336-9.

Li P, Wang HZ, Wang XQ, Wu YN. 1994. The blocking effect of phenolic acid on N-nitrosomorpholine formation in vitro. Biomed Environ Sci. 7(1):68-78.

Lin, Y.L., Hsu, Y.C., Chiu, Y.T., Huang, Y.T. 2008. Antifibrotic effects of a herbal combination regimen on hepatic fibrotic rats. Phytother Res. 22:69-76.

Lone, I.A., Kaur, G., Athar, M., Alam, M.S. 2007. Protective effect of *Rumex patientia* (English Spinach) roots on ferric nitrilotriacetate (Fe-NTA) induced hepatic oxidative stress and tumor promotion response. Food Chem Toxicol. 45:1821-9.

Lopatkin, N., Sivkov, A., Walther, C., Schlafke, S., Medvedev, A., Avdeichuk, J., Golubev, G., Melnik, K., Elenberger, N., Engelmann, U. 2005. Long-term efficacy and safety of a combination of sabal and urtica extract for lower urinary tract symptoms--a placebo-controlled, double-blind, multicentre trial. World J Urol. 23:139-46.

Luna-Herrera, J., Costa, M.C., Gonzalez, H.G., Rodrigues, A.I., Castilho, P.C., 2007. Synergistic antimycobacterial activities of sesquiterpene lactones from *Laurus* spp. J Antimicrob Chemother. 59,548-52.

Mahady, G.B., Pendland, S.L., Stoia, A., Hamill, F.A., Fabricant, D., Dietz, B.M., Chadwick, L.R., 2005. *In vitro* susceptibility of *Helicobacter pylori* to botanical extracts used traditionally for the treatment of gastrointestinal disorders. Phytother Res. 19,988-91.

Maksimović, Z., Dobrić, S., Kovacević, N., Milovanović, Z. 2004. Diuretic activity of Maydis stigma extract in rats. Pharmazie. 59:967-71.

Martineau, L.C., Couture, A., Spoor, D., Benhaddou-Andaloussi, A., Harris, C., Meddah, B., Leduc, C., Burt, A., Vuong, T., Mai Le, P., Prentki, M., Bennett, S.A., Arnason, J.T., Haddad, P.S. 2006. Anti-diabetic properties of the Canadian lowbush blueberry *Vaccinium angustifolium* Ait. Phytomedicine 13: 612-23.

Mauch, C., Bilkei, G., 2004. Strategic application of oregano feed supplements reduces sow mortality and improves reproductive performance--a case study. J Vet Pharmacol Ther. 27, 61-3.

McCune, L.M., Johns, T. 2002. Antioxidant activity in medicinal plants associated with the symptoms of diabetes mellitus used by the indigenous peoples of the North American boreal forest. J Ethnopharmacol 82:197-205.

Meeking, S. 2007. Treatment of acute adrenal insufficiency. Clin Tech Small Anim Pract. 22:36-9.

Meij, B.P., Mol, J.A., Bevers, M.M., Rijnberk, A. 1997. Alterations in anterior pituitary function of dogs with pituitary-dependent hyperadrenocorticism. J Endocrinol. 154:505-12.

Melzig, M.F. 2004. Goldenrod--a classical exponent in the urological phytotherapy. Wien Med Wochenschr. 154:523-7. Article in German.

Mencherini, T., Picerno, P., Scesa, C., Aquino, R. 2007. Triterpene, antioxidant, and antimicrobial compounds from *Melissa officinalis*. J Nat Prod. 70:1889-94.

Miceli, N., Taviano, M.F., Giuffrida, D., Trovato, A., Tzakou, O., Galati, E.M., 2005. Anti-inflammatory activity of extract and fractions from *Nepeta sibthorpii* Bentham. J Ethnopharmacol. 97,261-6.

Moon, M.K., Kang, D.G., Lee, J.K., Kim, J.S., Lee, H.S., 2006. Vasodilatory and anti-inflammatory effects of the aqueous extract of rhubarb via a NO-cGMP pathway. Life Sci. 78,1550-7.

Morel, A.F., Dias, G.O., Porto, C., Simionatto, E., Stuker, C.Z., Dalcol, I.I. 2006. Antimicrobial activity of extractives of *Solidago microglossa*. Fitoterapia 77: 453-5.

Muriel, P., Rivera-Espinoza, Y. 2007. Beneficial drugs for liver diseases. J Appl Toxicol. 28(2):93-103

Nakagiri, R., Hashizume, E., Kayahashi, S., Sakai, Y., Kamiya, T. 2003. Suppression by Hydrangeae Dulcis Folium of D-galactosamine-induced liver injury *in vitro* and *in vivo*. Biosci Biotechnol Biochem. 67:2641-3.

Nir, Y., Potasman, I., Stermer, E., Tabak, M., Neeman, I., 2000. Controlled trial of the effect of cinnamon extract on *Helicobacter pylori*. Helicobacter. 5,94-7.

Nomikos, T., Detopoulou, P., Fragopoulou, E., Pliakis, E., Antonopoulou, S. 2007. Boiled wild artichoke reduces postprandial glycemic and insulinemic responses in normal subjects but has no effect on metabolic syndrome patients. Nutrition Research 27: 741 – 749.

Nguyen TK, Obatomi DK, Bach PH. 2001. Increased urinary uronic acid excretion in experimentally-induced renal papillary necrosis in rats. Ren Fail. 23(1):31-42.

Oh, H., Kim, D.H., Cho, J.H., Kim, Y.C. 2004. Hepatoprotective and free radical scavenging activities of phenolic petrosins and flavonoids isolated from *Equisetum arvense*. J Ethnopharmacol. 95:421-4.

O'Mahony, R., Al-Khtheeri, H., Weerasekera, D., Fernando, N., Vaira, D., Holton, J., Basset, C., 2005. Bactericidal and anti-adhesive properties of culinary and medicinal plants against *Helicobacter pylori*. World J Gastroenterol. 11, 7499-507.

Omoruyi, F.O., McAnuff-Harding, M.A., Asemota, H.N. 2006. Intestinal lipids and minerals in streptozotocin-induced diabetic rats fed bitter yam (*Dioscorea polygonoides*) sapogenin extract. Pak J Pharm Sci. 19(4):269-75.

Ozkarsli, M., Sevim, H., Sen, A. 2008. *In vivo* effects of *Urtica urens* (dwarf nettle) on the expression of CYP1A in control and 3-methylcholanthrene-exposed rats. Xenobiotica 38:48-61.

Panossian, A., Wagner, H. 2005. Stimulating effect of adaptogens: An overview with particular reference to their efficacy following single dose administration. Phytother Res. 19: 819-38.

Papadopoulos, V., Widmaier, E.P., Amri, H., Zilz, A., Li, H., Culty, M., Castello, R., Philip, G.H., Sridaran, R., Drieu, K. 1998. *In vivo* studies on the role of the peripheral benzodiazepine receptor (PBR) in steroidogenesis. Endocr Res. 24:479-87.

Papiez M, Gancarczyk M, Bilińska B. 2002. The compounds from the hollyhock extract (*Althaea rosea* Cav. var. *nigra*) affect the aromatization in rat testicular cells in vivo and in vitro. Folia Histochem Cytobiol. 40(4):353-9.

Pari, L., KarthiKesan, K. 2007. Protective role of caffeic acid against alcohol-induced biochemical changes in rats. Fundamental and Clinical Pharmacology 21: 355- 361.

Park, E.J., Nan, J.X., Zhao, Y.Z., Lee, S.H., Kim, Y.H., Nam, J.B., Lee, J.J., Sohn, D.H. 2004. Water-soluble polysaccharide from *Eleutherococcus senticosus* stems attenuates fulminant hepatic failure induced by D-galactosamine and lipopolysaccharide in mice. Basic Clin Pharmacol Toxicol. 94:298-304.

Pereira, R.S., Sumita, T.C., Furlan, M.R., Jorge, A.O., Ueno, M. 2004. Antibacterial activity of essential oils on microorganisms isolated from urinary tract infection. Rev Saude Publica 38:326-8. Article in Portuguese.

Pereira, R.S., Sumita, T.C., Furlan, M.R., Jorge, A.O., Ueno, M., 2004. Antibacterial activity of essential oils on microorganisms isolated from urinary tract infection. Rev Saude Publica 38,326-8. Article in Portuguese.

Petlevski, R., Hadzija, M., Slijepcevic, M., Juretic, D., Petrik, J. 2003. Glutathione S-transferases and malondialdehyde in the liver of NOD mice on short-term treatment with plant mixture extract P-9801091. Phytother Res. 17:311-4.

Randhir, R., Shetty, K., 2007. Improved alpha-amylase and *Helicobacter pylori* inhibition by fenugreek extracts derived via solid-state bioconversion using *Rhizopus oligosporus*. Asia Pac J Clin Nutr. 16,382-92.

Salamci, E., Kordali, S., Kotan, R., Cakir, A., Kaya, Y., 2007. Chemical compositions, antimicrobial and herbicidal effects of essential oils isolated from Turkish *Tanacetum aucheranum* and *Tanacetum chiliophyllum* var. *chiliophyllum*. Biochemical Systematics and Ecology 35, 569-581.

Savino, F., Cresi, F., Castagno, E., Silvestro, L., Oggero, R. 2005. A randomized double-blind placebo-controlled trial of a standardized extract of *Matricariae recutita, Foeniculum vulgare* and *Melissa officinalis* (ColiMil) in the treatment of breastfed colicky infants. Phytother Res. 19(4):335-40.

Shimizu, M., Shiota, S., Mizushima, T., Ito, H., Hatano, T., Yoshida, T., Tsuchiya, T. 2001. Marked potentiation of activity of beta-lactams against methicillin-resistant *Staphylococcus aureus* by corilagin. Antimicrob Agents Chemother 45(11):3198-201.

Shrivastava, R., Cucuat, N., John, G.W. 2007. Effects of *Alchemilla vulgaris* and glycerine on epithelial and myofibroblast cell growth and cutaneous lesion healing in rats. Phytother Res. 21: 369-73.

Shrivastava, R., John, G.W. 2006. Treatment of aphthous stomatitis with topical *Alchemilla vulgaris* in glycerine. Clin Drug Investig. 26, 567-73.

Singh, G., Maurya, S., DeLampasona, M.P., Catalan, C.A., 2007. A comparison of chemical, antioxidant and antimicrobial studies of cinnamon leaf and bark volatile oils, oleoresins and their constituents. Food Chem Toxicol. 45,1650-61.

Singh, Y.N., Devkota, A.K., Sneeden, D.C., Singh, K.K., Halaweish, F. 2007. Hepatotoxicity potential of saw palmetto (*Serenoa repens*) in rats. Phytomedicine 14:204-8.

Speroni, E., Cervellati, R., Govoni, P., Guizzardi, S., Renzulli, C., Guerra, M.C. 2003. Efficacy of different *Cynara scolymus* preparations on liver complaints. J Ethnopharmacol. 86:203-11.

Stamatis, G., Kyriazopoulos, P., Golegou, S., Basayiannis, A., Skaltsas, S., Skaltsa, H., 2003. *In vitro* anti-*Helicobacter pylori* activity of Greek herbal medicines. J Ethnopharmacol. 88,175-9.

Steenkamp, V., Gouws, M.C., Gulumian, M., Elgorashi, E.E., van Staden, J. 2006. Studies on antibacterial, anti-inflammatory and antioxidant activity of herbal remedies used in the treatment of benign prostatic hyperplasia and prostatitis. J Ethnopharmacol. 103:71-5.

Thompson, R.C., Palmer, C.S., O'Handley, R., 2007. The public health and clinical significance of Giardia and Cryptosporidium in domestic animals. Vet J. 177(1):18-25.

Tunón, H., Olavsdotter, C., Bohlin, L. 1995. Evaluation of anti-inflammatory activity of some Swedish medicinal plants. Inhibition of prostaglandin biosynthesis and PAF-induced exocytosis. Journal of Ethnopharmacology 48: 61-76.

Turker, A.U., Usta, C., 2008. Biological screening of some Turkish medicinal plant extracts for antimicrobial and toxicity activities. Nat Prod Res. 22,136-46.

Uzun, E., Sariyar, G., Adsersen, A., Karakoc, B., Ötük, G., Oktayoglu, E., Pirildar, S. 2004. Traditional medicine in Sakarya province (Turkey) and antimicrobial activities of selected species. J Ethnopharmacol. 95:287-96.

van den Berg, A.J., Labadie, R.P., 1984. Anthraquinones, anthrones and dianthrones in callus cultures of *Rhamnus frangula* and *Rhamnus purshiana*. Planta Med. 50,449-51.

Vanisree, A.J., Sudha, N. 2006. Curcumin combats against cigarette smoke and ethanol-induced lipid alterations in rat lung and liver. Mol Cell Biochem. 288:115-23.

Varzi H.N., Esmailzadeh, S., Morovvati, H., Avizeh, R., Shahriari, A., Givi, M.E. 2007. Effect of silymarin and vitamin E on gentamicin-induced nephrotoxicity in dogs. J Vet Pharmacol Ther. 30:477-81.

Velazquez, D.V., Xavier, H.S., Batista, J.E., de Castro-Chaves, C. 2005. *Zea mays* L. extracts modify glomerular function and potassium urinary excretion in conscious rats. Phytomedicine 12:363-9.

Venkatesan, N., Punithavathi, D., Arumugam, V. 2000. Curcumin prevents adriamycin nephrotoxicity in rats. Br J Pharmacol. 129:231-4.

Verma, R.J., Asnani, V. 2007. Ginger extract ameliorates paraben induced biochemical changes in liver and kidney of mice. Acta Pol Pharm. 64:217-20.

Villar A, Gascó MA, Alcaraz MJ. Some aspects of the inhibitory activity of hypolaetin-8-glucoside in acute inflammation. J Pharm Pharmacol. 1987 Jul;39(7):502-7.

Villaseñor-García, M.M., Lozoya, X., Osuna-Torres, L., Viveros-Paredes, J.M., Sandoval-Ramírez, L., Puebla-Pérez, A.M. 2004. Effect of *Ginkgo biloba* extract EGb 761 on the nonspecific and humoral immune responses in a hypothalamic-pituitary-adrenal axis activation model. Int Immunopharmacol. 4:1217-22.

Vlahović, P., Cvetković, T., Savić, V., Stefanović, V. 2007. Dietary curcumin does not protect kidney in glycerol-induced acute renal failure. Food Chem Toxicol. 45:1777-82.

Watt, K., Christofi, N., Young, R. 2007.The detection of antibacterial actions of whole herb tinctures using luminescent *Escherichia coli*. Phytother Res. 21:1193-9.

Weckesser, S., Engel, K., Simon-Haarhaus, B., Wittmer, A., Pelz, K., Schempp, C.M., 2007. Screening of plant extracts for antimicrobial activity against bacteria and yeasts with dermatological relevance. Phytomedicine 14,508-16.

Wittschier N, Lengsfeld C, Vorthems S, Stratmann U, Ernst JF, Verspohl EJ, Hensel A. 2007. Large molecules as anti-adhesive compounds against pathogens. J Pharm Pharmacol. 59(6):777-86.

Wynn, S.G., Marsden, S.A. 2003. Manual of Natural Veterinary Medicine: Science and Tradition. Mosby: St Louis.

Xiao, B., Guo, J., Liu, D., Zhang, S., 2007. Aloe-emodin induces in vitro G2/M arrest and alkaline phosphatase activation in human oral cancer KB cells. Oral Oncol. 43,905-10.

Yamamoto, J., Yamada, K., Naemura, A., Yamashita, T., Arai, R. 2005. Testing various herbs for antithrombotic effect. Nutrition 21:580-7.

Yarnell, E. 2002. Botanical medicines for the urinary tract. World J Urol. 20:285-93

Ye, M., Han, J., Chen, H., Zheng, J., Guo, D., 2006. Analysis of phenolic compounds in rhubarbs using liquid chromatography coupled with electrospray ionization mass spectrometry. J Am Soc Mass Spectrom. 18,82-91.

Yoo, M.Y., Oh, K.S., Lee, J.W., Seo, H.W., Yon, G.H., Kwon, D.Y., Kim, Y.S., Ryu, S.Y., Lee, B.H., 2007. Vasorelaxant effect of stilbenes from rhizome extract of rhubarb (*Rheum undulatum*) on the contractility of rat aorta. Phytother Res 21,186-9.

Zeugswetter, F., Hoyer, M.T., Pagitz, M., Benesch, T., Hittmair, K.M., Thalhammer, J.G. 2007. The desmopressin stimulation test in dogs with Cushing's syndrome. Domest Anim Endocrinol. 34(3):254-60.

Zhang, H., Matsuda, H., Kumahara, A., Ito, Y., Nakamura, S., Yoshikawa, M. 2007a. New type of anti-diabetic compounds from the processed leaves of *Hydrangea macrophylla* var. *thunbergii* (Hydrangeae Dulcis Folium). Bioorg Med Chem Lett. 17:4972-6.

Zhang, J., Zhang, X., Lei, G., Li, B., Chen, J., Zhou, T. 2007b. A new phenolic glycoside from the aerial parts of *Solidago canadensis*. Fitoterapia 78: 69–71.

Zheng, W., Wang, S.Y., 2001. Antioxidant activity and phenolic compounds in selected herbs. J Agric Food Chem. 49,5165-70.

Zhou, H., Jiao, D., 1990. 312 cases of gastric and duodenal ulcer bleeding treated with 3 kinds of alcoholic extract rhubarb tablets. Zhong Xi Yi Jie He Za Zhi. 10,150-1, 131-2. [Article in Chinese]

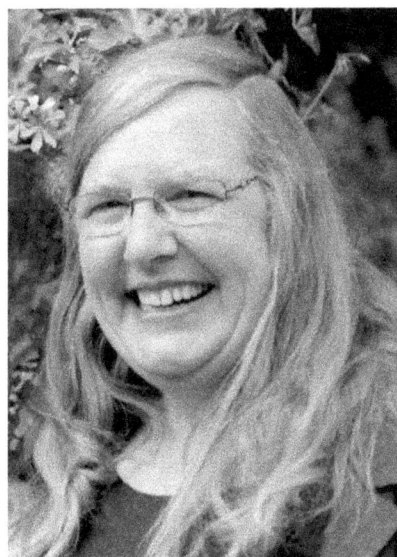

Nancy Turner is an ethnobotanist and Distinguished Professor in the School of Environmental Studies at the University of Victoria. She is also a Research Associate with the Royal British Columbia Museum and an Adjunct Professor in Geography, and at the University of Manitoba, Natural Resources Institute.

http://cahr.uvic.ca/featured/cahr-july-2011-researcher-of-the-month-dr-nancy-turner/

TABLE 7. PLANTS USED FOR KIDNEY, LIVER AND URINARY PROBLEMS IN PETS IN BRITISH COLUMBIA

Scientific name	Common name	Plant part used	Use
Alchemilla arvensis Lamk. (Rosaceae)	parsley piert	whole herb	kidney tonic
Althaea officinalis L. (Malvaceae)	marshmallow	root	ingredient in commercial kidney and blood pressure tea
Arctium lappa L. (Asteraceae)	burdock	roots	liver tonic
Arctostaphylos uva ursi L. (Ericaceae)	uva ursi	berry, leaf	ingredient in commercial kidney and blood pressure tea, spay related incontinence, cystitis, urinary problems
Berberis aquifolium Pursh. *Mahonia aquifolium* (Berberidaceae)	Oregon grape	root	spay related incontinence
Carum petroselinum	parsley		ingredient in kidney and blood pressure tea
Curcuma longa L. (Zingiberaceae)	turmeric	root	ingredient in commercial liver products
Cynara scolymus L. (Asteraceae)	artichoke	leaf	ingredient in purchased liver product A, tonic
Dioscorea villosa L. (Dioscoreaceae)	wild yam	root	ingredient in commercial liver products, Addison's disease
Eleutherococcus senticosus Maxim. (Araliaceae)	eleuthero root	root	Addison's disease, ingredient in commercial liver products
Equisetum palustre L. (Equisetaceae)	horsetail	aerial parts	ingredient in kidney and blood pressure tea
Eupatorium purpureum L., (Asteraceae)	gravel root	whole plant, roots	ingredient in kidney and blood pressure tea
Ginkgo biloba	ginkgo	leaf	Cushing's disease, hyperadrenocorticism
Glycyrrhiza glabra L. (Fabaceae)	licorice	root	Addison's disease, ingredient in commercial liver product A
Hydrangea arborescens L. (Hydrangeaceae)	hydrangea	root	kidney tonic
Hydrastis canadensis L. (Ranunculaceae)	goldenseal	root	ingredient in commercial kidney and blood pressure tea
Juniperus communis L. (Cupressaceae)	common juniper	berry	ingredient in commercial kidney and blood pressure tea, urinary problems
Melissa officinalis L. (Lamiaceae)	lemon balm	aerial parts	toner for urinary problems
P*etroselinum* crispum (P. Mill.) Nyman ex A.W. Hill (Apiaceae)	parsley	aerial parts	urinary problems
Rehmannia glutinosa (Gaertn.) Steud.	rehmannia	root	ingredient in purchased liver tonic A

(Gesneriaceae)			
Rosmarinus officinalis L. (Lamiaceae)	rosemary	leaf	ingredient in commercial liver tonic B
Rumex crispus L. (Polygonaceae)	curly dock	roots	liver support, urinary problems
Schisandra chinensis (Turcz.) Baill. (Schisandraceae)	schisandra	fruit	ingredient in commercial liver tonic B
Serenoa repens (Bartr.) Small (Arecaceae)	saw palmetto	fruit	benign hyperplasia & prostate support
Silybum marianum Gaertn. (Asteraceae)	milk thistle	seed	ingredient in commercial liver products A & B
Solidago virgaurea L., (Asteraceae)	goldenrod	aerial parts	ingredient in commercial kidney and blood pressure tea
Taraxacum officinale (L.) Weber (Asteraceae)	dandelion	root	ingredient in commercial liver product A
Urtica dioica L. (Urticaceae)	nettles	roots, leaves	kidney tonic, malformed kidneys, ingredient in kidney and blood pressure tea
Vaccinium macrocarpon Aiton (Ericaceae)	cranberry	fruit juice	urinary problems, cystitis
Vaccinium myrtillus L. (Ericaceae)	bilberry	leaves	urinary problems
Zea mays L. (Poaceae)	corn	Silk	cat straining to urinate, kidney tonic
Zingiber officinale Roscoe (Zingiberaceae)	ginger	Rhizome	ingredient in commercial kidney and blood pressure tea

TABLE 8. TREATMENTS AND DOSAGES FOR KIDNEY AND LIVER PROBLEMS IN PETS IN BRITISH COLUMBIA

Plant name	Condition	Tea preparation	Tincture preparation	Dosages
Arctium lappa	liver tonic	Decoction of 5 ml (1 tsp) of thinly-sliced, fresh or dried burdock root in 224 ml water		250 ml per 46 kg patient bodyweight put in the pet's food until healthy
Arctostaphylos uva-ursi	cystitis			
Melissa officinalis	toner for urinary problems			30 ml (2 tbsp) of the herb in 114 ml of boiling water per 11 to 14 kg patient bodyweight). given as the drinking water
Rumex crispus	urinary problems	250 ml water and 240 ml (1 cup) chopped, fresh or dried yellow dock root		60 ml (1/4 cup) of the liquid a day per 11 to 14 kg patient bodyweight for two days
Rumex crispus	liver problems		A 1:5 tincture was made in 50% alcohol. Or a 1:2 tincture of fresh root in 50% alcohol.	3 g of dried root. 1:5 Tincture: 15 drops /day of the tincture per 46 kg patient bodyweight. 1:2 tincture-10 drops /day per 46 kg patient bodyweight
Silybum marianum	liver problems			23 kg dog got ground milk thistle seed- 50 mg per 4.5 kgs twice a day. Broccoli and brussel sprouts were fed.
Vaccinium macrocarpon	urinary problems			100 – 200 mg powder for 4.5 kg cats and 300 mg for

				14 kg dogs three to four days a month (10 mg/0.5 kg patient bodyweight), given with food.
Vaccinium macrocarpon	cystitis in cats	put in the water or was given as a liquid drench		2 drops put on their nose
Zea mays	cats with bloody urine	60 ml (¼ cup) cut corn silk in 0.45 L of boiling water		
Zea mays	cats with bloody urine	chopped fresh corn silk was fed raw		

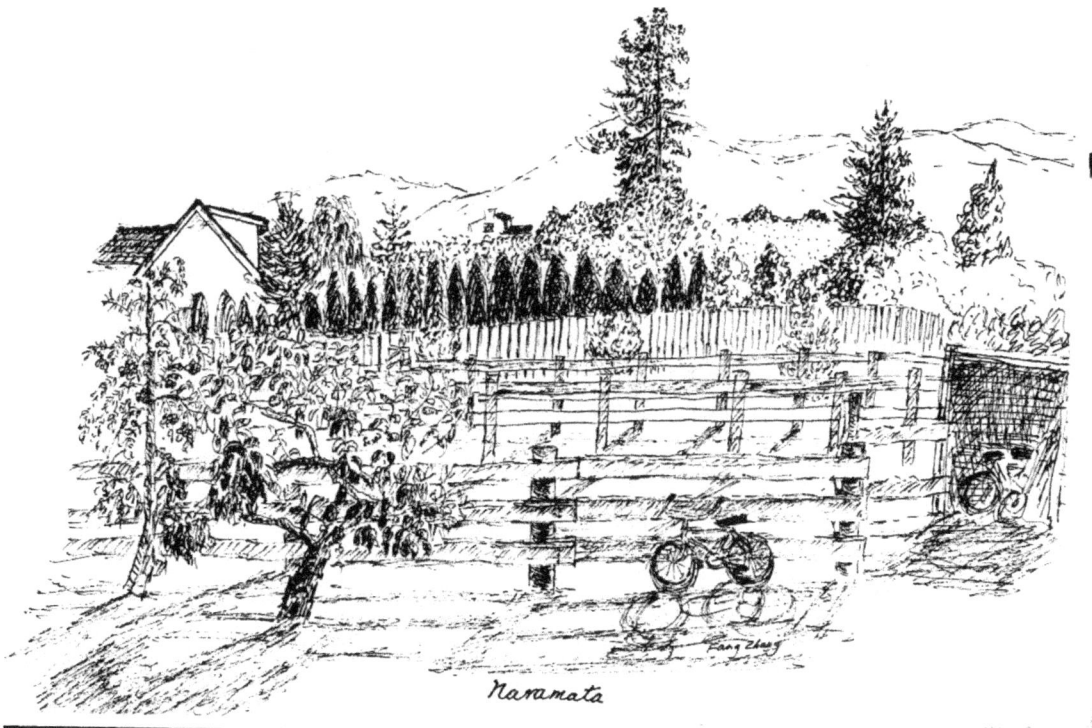

Naramata

TABLE 9. TREATMENTS FOR GASTROINTESTINAL PROBLEMS, CONSTIPATION AND MEGACOLON IN CATS AND DOGS IN BRITISH COLUMBIA

Scientific name	Common name	Plant part used	Use
Althaea officinalis (Malvaceae)	marshmallow	R	Mg, GP
Anethum graveolens (Apiaceae)	dill	L, F, S	GP
Arctium lappa (Asteraceae)	burdock	R	GP
Cetraria islandica (Parmeliaceae)	Iceland moss	Pl	GP
Cinnamomum zeylanicum Blume (Lauraceae)	cinnamon	B	GP
Coriandrum sativum (Apiaceae)	coriander	S, L, F	GP
Eugenia caryophyllus (Myrtaceae)	cloves	Fr	GP
Foeniculum vulgare (Apiaceae)	fennel	S	GP
Frangula purshiana (DC.) Cooper (Rhamnaceae)	cascara	B	Mg
Gentiana lutea (Gentianaceae)	gentian	R	GP
Glycyrrhiza glabra (Fabaceae)	licorice	R	Mg
Laurus nobilis (Lauraceae).	bay	L	GP
Nepeta cataria (Lamiaceae)	catnip	Ft	GP
Origanum vulgaris/ Origanum marjorana (Lamiaceae)	sweet majoram, oregano	Ap	GP
Rheum palmatum	rhubarb	Fs	Mg
Salvia officinalis (Lamiaceae)	sage	L	GP
Thymus vulgaris (Lamiaceae)	thyme	Ap	GP
Trigonella foenum-graecum (Leguminosae)	fenugreek	S	GP
Ulmus fulva (Ulmaceae)	slippery elm	B	Mg
Urtica dioica (Urticaceae)	nettles	Ap	GP
Zingiber officinalis (Zingiberaceae)	ginger	Rh	Mg

Key: L=leaves; S = seeds; F= flowers; M = moss; R = root; Fr = fruit; B = bark; Bp = bark powder; Hu = husks; Aerial parts = Ap; Rh = rhizome; Fresh stem = Fs; Flowering tops = Ft; Pl = plant; GP = gastrointestinal problems; Mg = megacolon,

TABLE 10. TREATMENT DETAILS FOR GASTROINTESTINAL PROBLEMS, CONSTIPATION AND EMESIS IN CATS AND DOGS IN BRITISH COLUMBIA

Medicinal plants	Plant parts	Disease, condition	Preparation and dose (tea, decoction)	Preparation and dose (tincture)
Althaea officinalis	R	irritable bowel, colitis and ulcers	30 ml (2 tbsp) water with 2 ml (½ tsp) parts.	
Anethum graveolens	L,S,F	GP	Tea made from 5 – 10 ml (1-2 tsp) crushed parts in 250 ml water for flatulence. 5 ml (1 tsp) daily per 11.4 kgs bodyweight orally with a syringe or in the drinking water	Tincture 1- 2 ml three times a day
Arctium lappa	R	GP	Decoction made of 5 ml (1 tsp) of thinly-sliced, fresh or dried root simmered in 236.8 ml water in a glass or ceramic pan. Give 250 ml in water or 125 in combination with nettles.	
Cetraria islandica	M	GP	Decoction 5 ml (1 tsp) parts in 250 ml water give 250 ml twice daily. 250 ml tea before meals per 45.5kg bodyweight	Tincture -1- 2 ml per 20 -25 kgs patient bodyweight three times a day orally or in the drinking water
Coriandrum sativum	F, L, S	GP	Tea made from 10 ml (2 tsp) crushed parts in 250 ml water	
Nepeta cataria	F	GP	5 – 10 ml (1 – 2 tsp) parts in 250 ml water. 1 tsp daily per 11.4 kgs bodyweight orally with a syringe or in the drinking water	
Origanum marjorana or *Origanum vulgaris*	F, L	GP	5 – 10 ml (1 - 2 tsp) sweet marjoram parts	
Plantago ovata	Hu, S	general constipation	250 ml of boiling water over 5 ml (1 tsp) of psyllium parts per 9 – 11 kgs bodyweight	
Rubus idaeus, R. strigosus	L, Fr	GP	5 – 10 ml (1 - 2 tsp) herb in 250 ml water. Dose is 1 tsp daily per 11.4 kgs bodyweight orally with a syringe or in the drinking water.	
Ascophyllum odosum, Laminaria		emesis (yellow bile)	A supplement with dehydrated oatmeal, carrots and seaweeds was fed to two Bichons at night to	

digitata			prevent emesis.	
Thymus vulgaris	L	GP	5 – 10 ml (1 - 2 tsp) herb in 250 ml water. Dose is 1 tsp daily per 11.4 kgs bodyweight orally with a syringe or in the drinking water.	
Ulmus fulva	Bp	irritable bowel, colitis and ulcers	60 ml (4 tbsp) of slippery elm bark powder per 55 kgs bodyweight in a little water twice a day. This is given orally with a syringe or in a bowl if essential fatty acids are added (½ to 1 tsp per 23 kgs).	
Ulmus fulva	Bp	food poisoning	1 ml (¼ tsp) of slippery elm bark powder1 capsule of activated charcoal, 2 ml (1/2 tsp) selenium and 4 ginger pills (or 1 tsp or 5 ml) per 18 kgs bodyweight.	

Key: L=leaves; S = seeds; F= flowers; M = moss; R = root; Fr = fruit; B = bark; Bp = bark powder; Hu = husks; GP = gastrointestinal problems

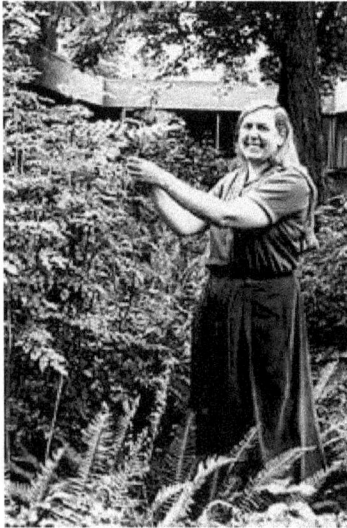

http://ring.uvic.ca/97oct17/Nancy%20_Turner.html

Ethnobotanist Dr. Nancy Turner (Environmental Studies)

TABLE 11. NON-EXPERIMENTAL VALIDATION OF PLANTS USED FOR MEGACOLON, URINARY, GASTROINTESTINAL, ENDOCRINOPATHIES AND HEPATIC DISEASES AND OTHER PROBLEMS IN CATS AND DOGS IN BRITISH COLUMBIA

Medicinal plant	Validation information	Reference	Validation
Alchemilla arvensis	Used in a kidney tonic in this research. The plant showed no inhibitory effect in a prostaglandin test but did show PAF-inhibiting activity. The active constituents in *A. vulgaris* include polyphenols, and its activities include inhibition of intercellular matrix degrading proteases, antioxidant and angioprotective activities. The plant contains tannins (gallic and ellagic acid), flavonoids (quercetin, luteolin) and proanthocyanidins.	Tunón et al., 1995; Shrivastava and John, 2006; Shrivastava et al., 2007	3
Althaea officinalis	An ingredient in a kidney/blood pressure tea given to pets. The plant contains butyric acid, chlorogenic acid, ferulic acid, quercetin, caffeic acid, uronic acid, salicylic acid and several other compounds. Caffeic acid at a dose of 12mg/kg when given to rats with alcohol decreased the activities of serum AST, ALT, ALP, GGT, bilirubin, urea and creatinine and restored creatine clearance. Liver damage was minimised. A dose of 6 mg/kg was less effective.	De Smet and D'Arcy, 1996; Duke, 2008	3
Althaea officinalis	A treatment for megacolon and gastrointestinal problems in pets. Marshmallow may interfere with hypoglycaemic therapy and so should not be fed to diabetic animals. *Althaea officinalis* has antibacterial activity against *E. coli*. It contains coumarins and phenolic acid.	De Smet and D'Arcy, 1996; Watt et al., 2007	3
Anethum graveolens	Dill was used for gastrointestinal problems in this study. A terpenoid in dill's essential oil has anti-bacterial activity. *A. graveolens* seed extracts have significant mucosal protective and antisecretory effects of the gastric mucosa in mice. Dill fruit has an antispasmodic effect on the smooth muscles of the gastrointestinal tract.	Cowan, 1999; Hosseinzadeh et al., 2002	3

Arctium lappa	A liver tonic for pets in this study. *Arctium lappa* improved hepatic outcome in rats fed liquid ethanol and injected with carbon tetrachloride, both histopathologically and using biochemical parameters. It also has free radical scavenging activity in rats similarly treated with carbon tetrachloride. Arctigenin, a lignan in *Arctium lappa*, has antioxidant, antimicrobial and anti-inflammatory activities. *Arctium lappa* also has moderate antibacterial and anticandidal activity.	Jellinek, and Maloney, 2005; Cho et al., 2004; Holetz et al., 2002	4
Arctostaphylos uva-ursi	In this research *Arctostaphylos uva-ursi* was used for urinary problems, spay related incontinence and cystitis. *Arctostaphylos uva-ursi* is a well-known urinary antiseptic and anti-adhesion herb. Aqueous extracts of *Arctostaphylos uva-ursi* increased urine flow in rats. An extract of *Arctostaphylos uva-ursi* significantly reduced the MICs of beta-lactam antibiotics, such as oxacillin and cefmetazole, against methicillin-resistant *Staphylococcus aureus*. The active compound, corilagin, showed a synergistic bactericidal action when added to the growth medium in combination with oxacillin. This herb should not be administered with any substances that cause acidic urine, such as ascorbic acid and ammonium chloride, as it will reduce the antibacterial effect.	Yarnell, 2002 ; Beaux et al., 1999 ; Shimizu et al., 2001 ; Blumenthal, 2000	4
Berberis vulgaris	*Berberis aquifolium* was used for spay related incontinence. The pharmacologic actions of berberine include inhibition of intestinal fluid accumulation and ion secretion, inhibition of smooth muscle contraction and reduction of inflammation. *In vitro* studies showed that berberine inhibited activator protein 1 (AP-1), a key transcription factor in inflammation and carcinogenesis. In another study berberine had a direct affect on several aspects of the inflammatory process. It exhibited dose-dependent inhibition of arachidonic acid release from cell membrane phospholipids, inhibition of thromboxane A2 from platelets, and inhibition of thrombus formation.	Anon,2000	4
Cetraria	Given to pets for gastrointestinal problems	Bucar et al.,	3

islandica	in this study. Iceland moss is traditionally used for treating inflammatory conditions such as gastritis, and has been considered safe. Five lichen compounds (a depsidone, aliphatic lactone, depside, dibenzofuran and anthraquinone) showed 5-lipoxygenase (5-LOX) inhibitory activity (anti-inflammatory). The constituent protolichesterinic acid has *in vitro* activity against *Helicobacter pylori* and against *Mycobacterium aurum*, a non-pathogenic organism with a similar sensitivity profile to *M. tuberculosis*.	2004; Ingólfsdóttir et al., 1998	
Cinnamomum zeylanicum	Used to treat pets with gastrointestinal problems in this study. *Cinnamomum zeylanicum* water extract had 85.5 ±1.3 HCV-PR inhibition (%) against hepatitis C virus (HCV) protease (PR). The methanol extract of cinnamon was effective against *Arcobacter butzleri*, *A. cryaerophilus*, and *A. skirrowii*, the zone of inhibition of the chloroform extract (30.9-mm and 41.2-mm) inhibition, was almost twice as large as that of the methanol extract for *A. butzleri* and *A. cryaerophilus*. *A. butzleri* and *A. cryaerophilus* are associated with enteritis in humans. *A. skirrowii* was isolated from a patient with chronic diarrhea. Cinnamon is also active against *C. jejuni* and *H. pylori*. One constituent, e-cinnamaldehyde has activity against *A. niger*, *A. flavus*, *A. ochraceus*, *F. graminearum*, *F. moniliforme*, *P. citrinum*, and *A. terreus*. It also has activity against *B. subtilis*, *S. aureus*, *B. cereus*, *E. coli*, *S. typhi* and *P. aeruginosa*. A cinnamon extract (80 mg /day) did not eradicate *H. pylori* in humans.	Hussein et al., 2000; Cervenka et al., 2006; Singh et al., 2007; Nir et al., 2000	3
Coriandrum sativum	Coriander was given to pets with gastrointestinal problems in this study. *Coriandrum sativum* seed extracts have a protective role against the deleterious effects of lipid metabolism in 1,2-dimethylhydraxin (DMH)-induced colon carcinogenesis in the rat. In another study coriander provided dose-dependent protection against the damaging action of ethanol and other necrotizing agents on	Chithra and Leelamma, 2000; Al-Mofleh et al., 2006	3

	the gastric mucosa of rats. Linalool and flavonoids in coriander are said to be the active constituents.		
Curcuma longa	Turmeric was an ingredient in commercial liver products given to pets. There is a strong correlation between antioxidant activity and antiinflammatory activities of curcuminoids. Curcumin can alleviate liver damage. Curcumin given intraperitoneally up-regulated HO-1 protein expression as well as activity. The induction of HO-1 expression by curcumin provides protection against hepatic damage associated with induced oxidative stress in rats. Curcumin can attenuate liver injury induced by diverse hepatotoxicants via multiple mechanisms. Curcumin administration increased several cytoprotective enzymes, especially in the liver.	Darshan and Doreswamy, 2004; Vanisree and Sudha, 2006; El-Ashmawy et al., 2006; Farombi et al., 2007	3
Cynara scolymus	Part of a purchased liver tonic in this study given to pets. Artichoke leaf (*Cynara scolymus*) contains cynarin (choleretic activity), natural phenolic antioxidants such as hydroxycinnamic acids and flavones. A commerical extract was effective in MDA levels in liver as well as in serum enzymes levels; the extract with the highest content in phenolic derivatives (GAE) exerted the major effect on bile flow and liver protection. The different extracts had good antioxidant capacity. Consumption of wild artichoke (*C. cardunculus*) by healthy subjects may protect them from hyperglycemia and insulin resistance	Duke, 1990; Speroni et al., 2003; Nomikos et al., 2007; Goñi et al., 2005	4
Dioscorea villosa	Wild yam root was used for liver problems and Addison's disease in this study. Yam tuber contains viscous mucilage composed of soluble glycoprotein, dietary fiber, and plant saponins (diosgenin) that may modulate lipid metabolism. Diosgenin is a steroidal saponin, also found in the root of wild yam (*Dioscorea villosa*). It is considered safe (GRAS). Bitter yam sapogenin extract or commercial diosgenin (1%) supplemented diets were fed to diabetic male Wistar rats for three weeks. Bitter yam sapogenin extract or commercial diosgenin did not significantly	Benghuzzi et al., 2003. Omoruyi et al., 2006; Chen et al., 2003; Hsu et al., 2007	4

	alter faecal magnesium, calcium, and zinc excretion but significantly decreased faecal sodium and potassium excretion. The absorption of iron was impaired by bitter yam sapogenin extract or commercial diosgenin during the first week of feeding. Bitter yam sapogenin extract or commercial diosgenin supplements significantly decreased intestinal lipids towards normal. Faecal lipids excreted was significantly higher in diabetic rats fed bitter yam sapogenin extract or commercial diosgenin for the three weeks period compared to the diabetic control group. *Dioscorea opposita* Thunb. rhizome extract can improve insulin resistance in rats receiving fructose-rich chow.		
Eleutherococcus senticosus	Pets were treated with *Eleutherococcus senticosus* for Addison's disease and it was an ingredient in commercial liver products. *E. senticosus* stems attenuate fulminant hepatic failure induced by D-galactosamine/ lipopolysaccharide in mice and the active ingredients are water-soluble polysaccharides in the stems. It protects mice from fulminant hepatic failure induced by GaIN/LPS by lowering tumour necrosis factor-alpha in serum and inhibiting apoptotic cell death of hepatocytes in liver.	Blumenthal, 2000, Anon, 2006. Park et al., 2004	4
Equisetum palustre	Kidney problems were treated with *Equisetum telmateia*. The petroleum extract had an MIC value of 39.1 µg/ml against *Staphylococcus epidermis*. *Equisetum arvense* has demonstrated hypoglycaemic and diuretic activity. The hydroalchoholic extract of stems of *Equisetum arvense* produced an antinociceptive effect and anti-inflammatory effects. The anti-inflammatory effects may be due to beta-sitosterol, campesterol and isofucosterol. The flavonoid isoquercitrin has anti-oxidant effects. A standardized extract from horsetail increased hippuric acid, the glycine conjugate of benzoic acid, in the urine of 11 volunteers.	Uzun et al., 2004, Gurbuz et al., 2002; Do Monte et al., 2004; Graefe and Veit, 1999;	3
Eugenia caryophyllus, Syn. *Syzygium aromaticum*	Pets were given cloves for gastrointestinal problems. The presence of compounds with	Ghayur et al., 2006; Chaieb et al., 2007	4

	spasmolytic and calcium antagonist activity may be responsible for the medicinal use of *Syzygium samarangense* in diarrhoea. The essential oil isolated from the buds of *Eugenia caryophyllata* is active against a large number of other bacteria: *Listeria monocytogenes*, *S. enterica*, *C. jejuni*, *S. enteritidis*, *E. coli* and *S. aureus* . clove oil showed activity against 32 multi-resistant *Staphylococcus epidermidis* strains with an inhibition zone of >16 mm. The oil was also active against 26 strains of *S. epidermidis* isolated from dialysis fluids, three human pathogenic Gram positive cocci, two Gram negative bacilli and one Gram positive bacillus (diameter of inhibition zone: 11–15 mm). It was ineffective against *P. aeruginosa*.		
Eupatorium purpureum	A kidney and blood pressure tea included *Eupatorium purpureum*. Cistifolin from the antirheumatic herb, gravel root (rhizome of *Eupatorium purpureum*), showed activity both in *in vitro* and *in vivo* models of inflammation.	Habtemariam, 2001,	3
Foeniculum vulgare	*Foeniculum vulgare* were used to treat gastrointestinal problems in pets. Smooth Move herbal tea, when added to the standard treatment regimen for nursing home residents with chronic constipation, increased the average number of bowel movements compared to the addition of a placebo tea (20 mg per cup Sennosides A & B (from senna leaf), Licorice Root, Fennel Seed, Orange Peel, Cinnamon Bark, Coriander Seed, Ginger Rhizome, Natural Orange Flavor). Colic in breastfed infanst improves within 1 week of treatment with an extract based on *Matricariae recutita*, *Foeniculum vulgare* and *Melissa officinalis*.	Bub et al., 2006; Savino et al., 2005	4
Frangula purshiana / *Rhamnus purshiana*	Megacolon in cats is treated with cascara bark. The glycosides of emodin, emodinanthrone and aloe-emodin were found in the freeze dried bark of *Rhamnus purshiana*.	van den Berg and Labadie, 1984	4
Gentiana lutea	Gentian roots were used for digestive problem in pets. The methanolic extracts of the aerial parts and the roots of *G. scabra* both have certain hepatoprotective effects on acute liver injury models.	Jiang and Xue, 2005; Aktay et al., 2000; Weckesser et al., 2007;	4

	Gentiana olivieri flowering plant showed hepatoprotective effects in rats. *Gentiana lutea* showed antimicrobial activity only against *Streptococcus pyogenes*. *Gentiana lutea* (roots), had antimicrobial activity (MIC of 100 µg/mL)against the gram-negative bacterium *Helicobacter pylori* (HP), identified as the primary etiological factor associated with the development of gastritis and peptic ulcer disease.	Mahady et al., 2005	
Ginkgo biloba	Ginkgo was used for Cushing's disease in our research. Ginkgolide B (normally obtained from the inner root bark) shortens the half-life of cortisol produced by the adrenals. It has been shown to have a regulatory effect on glucocorticoid levels. On rat tissue its inhibitory effect was limited to the adrenal cortex, corticosterone levels were decreased but aldosterone levels did not change. *Ginkgo biloba* extract also has immunostimulatory activity.	Papadopoulos et al., 1998; Wynn and Marsden, 2003; Amri et al., 2003; Villaseñor-García et al., 2004	4
Glycyrrhiza glabra	Licorice was used for megacolon in cats. Licorice was used for Addison's disease and was present in commercial liver products. Stronger neominophagen C (SNMC) is a Japanese preparation that contains 0.2% glycyrrhizin, 0.1% cysteine, and 2% glyceine. SNMC acts as an anti-inflammatory or cytoprotective drug. Glabridin was more active against Gram-positive bacterial strains than Gram-negative (*S. aureus, S. epidermidis, S. mutans, B. subtilis, E. faecalis, K. pneumoniae, S. typhi, Y. enterocolitica, E. aerogens* and *E. coli*).	Dhiman and Chawla, 2005; Gupta et al., 2008	4
Hydrangea arborescens	Hydrangea formed one ingredient in a purchased kidney tonic used for pets. The fermented and dried leaves of *Hydrangea macrophylla* SER. var. *thunbergii* MAKINO, suppressed D-galactosamine-induced liver injury by 85.2% when added to the diet at 1% and fed to rats for fifteen days. The hepatoprotective effect was more potent than that of a milk thistle extract and turmeric powder. The water-ethanol extract was active suggesting that the active compounds are lipophilic. Hydrangenol, phyllodulcin, thunberginol A,	Nakagiri et al., 2003; Zhang et al., 2007a	4

	and hydrangeaic acid from the processed leaves of *H. macrophylla* var. *thunbergii* promoted adipogenesis in 3T3-L1 cells. Hydrangenol significantly lowered blood glucose and free fatty acid levels 2 weeks after its administration at a dose of 200 mg/kg/d.		
Hydrastis canadensis	Goldenseal was used for urinary problems in pets. Berberine extracts and decoctions have demonstrated significant antimicrobial activity against a variety of organisms including bacteria, viruses, fungi, protozoans and chlamydia. The predominant clinical uses of berberine include bacterial diarrhea. Goldenseal can modulate the antigen-specific immune response, by enhancing the acute primary IgM response.	Anon, 2000	4
Juniperus communis	Juniper was used for kidney problems in pets. The aqueous ethanol extract of *Juniperus communis* (bark) showed pancreatic lipase inhibitory activity. The hydro-alcoholic extracts of branches of *Juniperus sabina* showed inhibitory activity against MDA-MB-468.	Kim and Kang, 2005; Madari and Jacobs, 2004.	3
Laurus nobilis	Bay leaves were used for gastrointestinal problems in pets. Sesquiterpene lactones, costunolide and dehydrocostuslactone, were the compounds responsible for the antimycobacterial activity against *Mycobacterium tuberculosis* H37Rv with MICs of 6.25 and 12.5 mg/L, respectively.	Luna-Herrera et al., 2007	3
Melissa officinalis	*Melissa officinalis* was used for urinary problems in pets. Major bacteriostatic effects were exerted against Gram-positive bacteria, *S. aureus* and *S. epidermidis*, by rosmarinic acid (MIC 0.12 mg/mL) and against *B. spizizenii* (MIC 0.5 mg/mL) by both of the dried leaf extracts EtOH-H2O (1:1), and *n*-BuOH. In the case of Gram-negative bacteria, yeasts, and molds the MICs were greater than 2.0 mg/mL. No antimicrobial effect was observed for rosmarinic acid at lower concentrations (5–250 μg/mL) in previous work. Rosmarinic acid is the major	Uzun et al., 2004; Savino et al., 2006; Mencherini et al., 2007	3

	bioactive compound present in *Melissa* extracts.		
Nepeta cataria	Catnip was used for gastrointestinal problems in this study. Extracts of *Nepeta atlantica* and *Nepeta tuberosa* contain iridoids and a lupane triterpine. The above species have analgesic activity. *Nepeta caesarea* showed significant analgesic activity, besides marked sedation, which was also blocked by naloxone, indicating involvement of opioid receptors but excluding mu-opioid receptors. The main antinociceptive component of the plant is nepetalactone. Anti-bacterial, fungicidal and anti-viral are attributed to nepetalactones (iridoids) found in several *Nepeta* species. *Nepeta cataria* L., *N. grandiflora* M.B., *N. mussinii* Spreng., *N. pannonica* L., and *Nepeta* x *faassenii* Berg., all contain the medicinally useful compounds ursolic and oleanolic acids.	Bouidida et al., 2006; Aydin et al., 1998; Calixto et al., 2000; Miceli et al., 2005; Janicsák et al., 2006.	3
Origanum vulgaris/ Origanum marjorana	Sweet marjoram and oregano were given to pets with gastrointestinal problems. *Origanum* x *majoricum* and *Origanum vulgare* ssp. *Hirtum* have high phenolic contents, including the anti-inflammatory rosmarinic acid. A commercial supplement contains the dried leaf and flower of *Origanum vulgare*, enriched with 500 g/kg cold-pressed essential oils of the leaf and flower of *Origanum vulgare*, 60-mg carvacrol and 55-mg thymol/kg. 43 oregano treated farrowing groups of 28–30 sows each (2117 sows of average parity of 2.98 ± 0.39) had fewer gastrointestinal problems than the control group.	Zheng and Wang, 2001; Mauch and Bilkei, 2004; Chun et al., 2005	4
Petroselinum crispum	Urinary problems in pets are treated with parsley. There is evidence for the diuretic effect of parsley (*Petroselinum crispum*). Rats offered an aqueous parsley seed extract to drink, eliminated a significantly larger volume of urine per 24 h as compared to when they were drinking water. Other experiments using an *in situ* kidney perfusion technique demonstrated a significant increase in urine flow rate with parsley seed extract. The mechanism of action of parsley seems to be mediated	Kreydiyyeh and Usta, 2002	4

	through an inhibition of the Na+-K+ pump that would lead to a reduction in Na+ and K+ reabsorption leading thus to an osmotic water flow into the lumen, and diuresis.		
Rehmannia glutinosa	Rehmannia glutinosa is found in purchased liver preparations used for pets. Alone and in combination with Astragalus it produced improved proteinuria, hematuria and renal function.	Geraghty, 2000; Kang et al., 2005	4
Rheum palmatum	Rhubarb was used to treat megacolon in cats. Medical results for Rheum rhaponticum show delayed disease progression; low serum cholesterol and triglycerides and significant improvement on proteinuria and severity of glomerulosclerosis of remnant kidney Aloe-emodin is a natural anthraquinone compound from the root and rhizome of Rheum palmatum. Piceatannol may be the major mediator responsible for the vasorelaxing properties of the rhizome extract of Rheum undulatum and the vasorelaxant effects of the piceatannol may be mediated via endothelium-dependent nitric oxide signaling pathway. Six rhubarb species, (Rheum officinale, R. palmatum, and R. tanguticum) and unofficial (R. franzenbachii, R. hotaoense, and R. emodi), had a total of 107 phenolic compounds. These compounds include sennosides, anthraquinones, stilbenes, glucose gallates, naphthalenes, and catechins. Sennoside A, which is considered the major purgative component of rhubarb, was only detected in R. officinale, while its close isomers were observed in R. palmatum and R. tanguticum. The predominant anthraquinone glycosides in R. officinale were found to be rhein 8-O-glucoside and emodin 1-O-glucoside, whereas those in R. palmatum and R. tanguticum were rhein 1-O-glucoside and emodin 8-O-glucoside.	Geraghty, 2000; Xiao et al., 2007; Yoo et al., 2007; Ye et al., 2007; Moon et al., 2006; Zhou and Jiao, 1990	4
Rosmarinus officinalis	Rosmarinus officinalis is an ingredient in commercial liver preparations used for pets. Rosemary (Rosmarinus officinalis) showed significant antithrombotic activity in vitro and in vivo. Both water and alcohol	Yamamoto et al., 2005; Amin and Hazma, 2005; Galisteo et al., 2006	4

	extracts of *Rosmarinus officinalis* have hepatoprotective effects against CCL4-induced liver damage. The liver protectant effects were attributed to antioxidant compounds in RO water extract (rosmarinic acid, diterpenoids like carnosic acid, carnosol, rosmanol and epirosmanol, carotenoids and alpha-tocopherol. A related plant *Rosmarinus tomentosus*, protected rat liver in an experimental model of cirrhosis.		
Rumex crispus	*Rumex crispus* is used for liver support and urinary problems in pets. Crude extracts of leaves of *Rumex nervosus* and the root of *Rumex abyssinicus* have antibacterial activity against *Streptococcus pyogenes* and *Staphylococcus aureus* and activity against Coxsackie virus B3. The methanol extract of the entire plant in Saudi Arabia possessed no activity against *E. coli, P. vulgaris, S. aureus* and *P. aeruginosa* and *C. albicans*. A similar extract of the leaves of the Mexican species showed weak activity against *E. coli, P. aeruginosa, S. aureus, Bacillus subtilis* and *C. albicans*. The 50% methanol of the flowers and leaves of the Nigerian species showed antibacterial activity against *B. subtilis, E. coli, Proteus* species, *P. aeruginosa* and *S. aureus*. Roots of *R. patientia* have significant antioxidant, hepatoprotective and antihyperproliferation properties.	Getie et al., 2003; Lone et al., 2007	4
Salvia officinalis	Gastrointestinal problems in pets are treated with sage. *Salvia officinalis*, L. showed enhanced inhibitory activity against bacterial strains derived from 100 urine samples taken from subjects diagnosed with urinary tract infection living in the community. The extract showed 100% efficiency against *Klebsiella* and *Enterobacter* species, 96% against *Escherichia coli*, 83% against *Proteus mirabilis*, and 75% against *Morganella morganii*.	Pereira et al., 2004	4
Serenoa repens	Saw palmetto is traditionally used for benign hyperplasia and prostate support and has this use for pets. Extracts from the fruits of saw palmetto (*Sabal serrulata*, syn. *Serenoa repens*)	Koch et al., 2001; Dreikorn, 2002	4

	and the roots of stinging nettle (*Urtica dioica*) are the most commonly used. Short-term randomised trials and some metaanalyses in the recent literature suggest clinical efficacy and good tolerability for extracts from *Serenoa repens* and also *Pygeum africanum*, products with high concentrations of beta-sitosterol, and pumpkin seeds. Studies have claimed that the efficacy of an extract from *S. repens* is comparable to that of finasteride and alpha-blockers.		
Schisandra chinensis	An incredient in a commercial liver tonic used for pets.

Schisandra (*Schisandra chinensis*) is a plant adaptogen or compound that increases the ability of an organism to adapt to environmental factors and to avoid damage from such factors. The SAS-mediated stimulating effects of single doses of adaptogens derived from *Rhodiola rosea*, *Schizandra chinensis* and *Eleutherococcus senticosus* were reviewed. The active principles of the three plants that exhibit single dose stimulating effects are glycosides of phenylpropane- and phenylethane-based phenolic compounds such as salidroside, rosavin, syringin and triandrin, the latter being the most active. Male Sprague-Dawley rats (n = 8–12 per group) were divided into the control, CCl4, CCl4 + silymarin (0.35%), CCl4 + low-dose herbal extract (0.24% of *Ginkgo biloba*, *Panax ginseng*, and *Schizandra chinensis* extract at 1:1:1; LE), and CCl4 + high-dose herbal extract (1.20% of the same herbal extract; HE) groups. Silymarin or herbal extract was orally given to rats a week before chronic intraperitoneal injection with CCl4 for 6 weeks. The high dose herbal extract improved hepatic antioxidant capacity through enhancing catalase activity and glutathione redox status, but the low-dose herbal extract inhibited liver fibrosis through decreasing hepatic TGF-β1 level in rats with CCl4-induced liver injury. | Panossian and Wagner, 2005; Chang et al., 2007 | 4 |
| *Silybum marianum* | Milk thistle was found in commercial liver products given to pets.

Silybum marianum and its derivatives have been used for centuries for the treatment | Boerth and Strong, 2002; Lieber et al., 2003; Ball and Kowdley, 2005; | 4 |

	of liver disease. The hepatoprotective action of silymarin, the active principle extracted from the fruit of *Silybum marianum* (L.) Gaertn., in animals (dogs, rabbits, rats, mice) intoxicated with phalloidine has been shown, both after protective and curative treatment. A dose of 15 mg/kg of silymarin protected every animal when given 60 min before the toxin. After 30 min its curative effect is negligible. *Silybum marianum* and its derivatives were shown to be safe. Silymarin did not reduce mortality in that studyand did not improve biochemistry and histology among patients with chronic liver disease. Oral administration of silybin in a phosphatidylcholine complex (phytosome) to dogs resulted in greater bioavailability of silybin compared with standard silymarin extract.	Desplaces et al., 1975; Dhiman and Chawla, 2005; Filburn et al., 2007	
Solidago canadensis	Goldenrod was used for urinary problems in pets. In European phytotherapy *Solidago canadensis* were used to treat chronic nephritis, cystitis, urolithiasis, rhematism and as an antiphlogistic. Compounds found in the plant include flavonoids, sesquiterpenes, diterpenes, triterpenes, saponins and a phenolic glycoside. Assessment of peroxyl radical scavenging activity showed *Solidago canadensis* extracts were greater than green tea, ascorbic acid and Trolox.	Zhang et al 2007b; McCune and Johns, 2002	3
Taraxacum officinale	Dandelions were given to pets for liver problems. The European Scientific Cooperative on Phytotherapy (ESCOP) recommends dandelion root (*Taraxacum officinale*) for kidney and liver problems, indigestion and loss of appetite. The German Commission E authorizes the use of combination products containing dandelion root and herb for biliary abnormalities, appetite loss, dyspepsia, and for stimulation of diuresis (urine flow). *Taraxacum officinalis* leaves contain potassium that replaces any lost from the body.	Petlevski et al., 2003; NSRC, 2004; Hoffman, 2003	4
Thymus vulgaris	Thyme leaves were used in teas for pets with gastrointestinal problems. Thyme (*Thymus vulgaris*) essential oil	Hersch-Martinez et al., 2005; Bonjar, 2004;	4

	showed high and broad antibacterial activity against prevalent pathogenic bacteria 189 Gram (-) and 135 Gram (+) strains in Mexico that were isolated from severely infected pediatric patients. *In vitro* anticandidal activity of the methanol extracts of *Thymus vulgaris* was evaluated at a 20 mg/ml concentration against Clotrimazole-resistant *Candida albicans*. *Thymus vulgaris* had a MIC of 0.62 mg/ml.		
Trigonella foenum-graecum	Fenugreek seeds were used for gastrointestinal problems in pets. Fenugreek is not a superoxide scavenger. Fenugreek may have hypo-cholesterolemic activity, and contains large amounts of the unconventional amino acid 4-hydroxy-isoleucine, which, along with its derivatives, is being developed as a novel antidiabetic molecule.	Langmead, 2002; Craig, 1999; Martineau et al., 2006	3
Ulmus fulva	*Ulmus fulva* were used for megacolon in cats. Slippery elms (*Ulmus rubra*, *Ulmus fulva*) were used to treat inflammatory bowel disease and its demulcent effect on mucosal membranes is recognised by the FDA. Slippery elm can be used in a combination formula with marshmallow root, indigo root (*Baptista tinctoria*), cranesbill and agrimony.	Langmead, 2002; Bock, 2000; De Smet and D'Arcy, 1996	3
Urtica dioica	Used for kidney problems in pets. The efficacy and tolerability of a fixed combination of 160 mg sabal fruit (burdock) extract WS 1473 and 120 mg urtica root extract WS 1031 per capsule (PRO 160/120) was investigated in elderly, male patients suffering from lower urinary tract symptoms (LUTS) caused by benign prostatic hyperplasia in a prospective multicenter trial in 257 patients (127 and 126 were evaluable for efficacy). Using the International Prostate Symptom Score (I-PSS), patients treated with PRO 160/120 had a higher total score reduction after 24 weeks of double-blind treatment than the placebo group. This applied to obstructive as well as to irritative symptoms, and to patients with moderate or severe symptoms at baseline. PRO 160/120 was clearly superior to the placebo for the amelioration of LUTS as measured by the	Koch et al., 2001; Petlevski et al., 2003; Lopatkin et al., 2005; Blumenthal, 2000; Ozkarsli et al., 2008	4

	I-PSS. *Urtica urens* can protect the body against environmental toxins.		
Urtica dioica	Nettles were given to pets with gastrointestinal problems.

Urtica dioica leaves had good inhibitory activity against *S. pyogenes*, *S. aureus* and *S. epidermidis*. A leaf infusion of *Urtica dioica* L. (2.5 g dry plant leaves infused in 1 L boiled water) protected rats that were given the chemical carcinogen trichloroacetic acid. | Turker and Usta, 2008; Celik and Tuluce, 2007 | 4 |
| *Vaccinium macrocarpon* | Bilberry leaves were used to treat pets with urinary problems.

Cranberry was used for urinary problems. Extracts of *Vaccinium angustifolium* possess insulin-like and glitazone-like activities and show anti-diabetic effects in pancreatic beta cells. Foliage of huckleberry (*Vaccinium* spp.) is fairly high in carotene, manganese, and energy. Bilberry extract protected against KBrO3-induced kidney damage, the active constituents may be anthocyanins. | Martineau et al., 2006; Petlevski et al., 2003; Acuña et al., 2002; Bao et al., 2008 | 4 |
| *Zea mays* | As for humans, corn silk was used for urinary problems in pets.

Studies have shown *in vivo* diuretic and hypotensive activity. Corn silk contains amines, fixed oils, saponins, tannins, bitter glycosides, allantoin, cryptoxanthin, flavone and phytosterols including beta-sitosterol and stigmasterol. The last two compounds are known to have antiinflammatory activity *in vivo* and may have a beneficial effect in treating prostate problems. | Habtemariam, 1998; Maksimović et al., 2004; Velazquez et al., 2005 | 4 |
| *Zingiber officinale* | Pets with urinary problems were treated with ginger.

The rhizome of ginger contains curcumin in addition to a dozen phenolic compounds known as gingerols and diarylheptanoids. These compounds possess significant antioxidant activity. The ethanol extract of *Z. officinale* alone and in combination with vitamin E provided significant protection against cisplatin-induced nephrotoxicity in rats which was evident from the lowered serum urea and creatinine levels. However the concentration of urea and creatinine in the *Z. officinale* treated groups were not | Craig, 1999; Bub et al., 2006; Ajith et al., 2007; Verma and Asnani, 2007 | 4 |

	normalized even in the 500 mg/kg treated group. The nephroprotection exhibited by *Z. officinale* can be correlated with its GST stimulating activity in the kidneys (the glutathione-s-transferase (GST) group of enzymes plays a major role in the detoxification pathway). Ginger may also protect the liver of mice from damage.		
Zingiber officinale	Pets with megacolon are treated with ginger. Ginger contains compounds (gingerdiones and shogaols) that have pharmacological properties mimicking dual-acting non-steroidal antiinflammatory drugs (NSAIDs) in intact human leukocytes *in vitro*, with fewer side effects. Ginger (and some of its constituents) is effective against cytokines synthesized and secreted at sites of inflammation. Smooth Move herbal tea contains ginger rhizome and increased the average number of bowel movements in a nursing home study. The active constituents of ginger (gingerols) had *in vitro* activity against *Helicobacter pylori*.	Craig, 1999; Bub et al., 2006; Ali et al., 2008	4

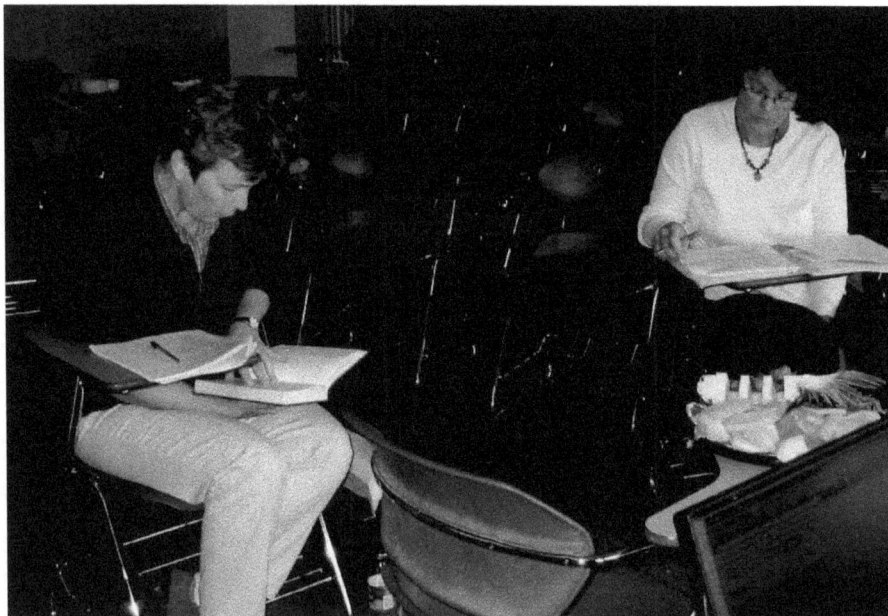

MEDICINAL PLANTS USED FOR SKIN PROBLEMS AND ALLERGIES IN PETS IN BRITISH COLUMBIA, CANADA

Abstract

Research conducted in 2003/2004 documented and validated (in a non-experimental way) ethnoveterinary medicines used in British Columbia (B.C.), Canada.

Interviews were conducted with 60 participants who were organic farmers or holistic medicinal/veterinary practitioners. This chapter reports on the medicinal plants used to treat skin problems in pets.

The plants used for skin problems are: *Aesculus hippocastanum*, *Aloe vera*, *Arctium lappa*, *Taraxacum officinale*, *Echinacea purpurea*, *Calendula officinalis*, *Cupressus sempervirens*, *Equisetum palustre*, *Galium aparine*, *Hydrastis canadensis*, *Hypericum perforatum*, *Plantago major*, *Thymus vulgaris*, *Rosmarinus officinalis*, *Rumex crispus*, *Stellaria media*, *Symphytum officinalis*, *Thuja occidentalis*, *Trigonella foenum-graecum* and *Urtica dioica*. Inhalant atopic dermatitis was treated with *Mahonia aquifolium*, *Glycyrrhiza glabra*, *Silybum marianum*, *Arctium lappa* and *Urtica dioica*. *Arctium lappa*, *Urtica dioica* and *Verbascum thapsus* are used for allergies. The development of holistic antiseptics and antimicrobial agents for the treatment of skin infections is increasingly important to deal with antibiotic-resistant bacteria.

Keywords: ethnoveterinary medicine, pets, British Columbia, skin problems, inhalant atopic dermatitis, allergies

This chapter focuses on the ethnoveterinary remedies used for skin problems (abscesses, wounds, yeast infections, burns and dermatitis) and allergies in pets in British Columbia.

Canine atopic dermatitis is an inflammatory and pruritic allergic skin disease linked to environmental allergens and makes dogs susceptible to secondary bacterial and yeast infections, especially to *Staphylococci* species (Nagle et al., 2001; Simou et al., 2005). Holistic treatments have been sought because of the side effects of glucocorticoids, the conventional treatment for this ailment (Saevik et al., 2004). Some mucilaginous herbs have been proposed as corticosteroid-sparing agents: flax (*Linum usitatissimum*), fenugreek (*Trigonella foenum graecum*), plantain (*Plantago* spp.), heartsease (*Viola tricolor*), marshmallow (*Althaea officinalis*), mulberry (*Morus* spp.), mullein (*Verbascum thapsus*), licorice (*Glycyrrhiza uralensis*), peony (*Paeonia lactiflora*), Rehmannia (*Rehmannia glutinosa*) and slippery elm (*Ulmus rubra*) (Sheehan et al., 1995; Millikan, 2003). Inclusions recommended in shampoos for pruritus are oatmeal (*Avena sativa*), *Aloe vera*, tea tree oil (*Melaleuca alternifolia*), and witch hazel (*Hamamelis virginiana*) (Wynn and Chalmers, 2002).

2. Materials and methods

The methods used in the research are described in the introductory chapter.

3. Results

The veterinarians who participated in the research were all small animal practitioners and all used standardized products. Table 12 lists the ethnoveterinary plants used to treat skin problems and allergies in pets. More details of the plant administration and preparation are given below under categories of ailments.

Treatment for abscesses

120

Cats and dogs with abscesses are treated with cultivated goldenseal (*Hydrastis canadensis*) and myrrh (*Commiphora molmol*). Dried leaves of goldenseal (3 grams) and 3 grams myrrh are infused for ½ hour in 475 ml of water. The infusion was dripped onto the cleaned wound for three days. Alternatively an infusion was made of 1 ml (1 tsp) of the combined herbs below in 475 ml olive oil and put on the food twice daily (per 12.5 kg patient bodyweight): comfrey (*Symphytum officinalis*), calendula (*Calendula officinalis*), plantain (*Plantago major*) and mullein (*Verbascum thapsus*). One drop of tincture of goldenseal in 10 drops (0.5 ml) of water was also given orally, three times daily, per 57kg patient bodyweight.

Ethnoveterinary treatment for skin problems, burns and wounds

The internal gel from the cut leaf of *Aloe vera* is used for skin regeneration. Skin problems are also treated with a purchased calendula ointment that also contained goldenseal (*Hydrastis canadensis*), *Echinacea* spp., horse chestnut (*Aesculus hippocastanum*), rosemary (*Rosmarinus officinalis*), thyme (*Thymus vulgaris*), fenugreek seeds (*Trigonella foenum-graecum*) and cypress (*Cupressus sempervirens*).

A purchased tincture of goldenseal (*Hydrastis canadensis*) (diluted 1:1 with sterile water or saline solution) is used as a disinfectant and for external cleansing. A decoction of common horsetail (*Equisetum arvense*) was made with 5 g (1 tsp) dried horsetail (or 3g fresh horsetail) for each 240 ml of water (or infusion with 240 ml of boiling water to each 8 grams (2 tsp) of dried silica-containing horsetail plant) and applied to abscesses.

A commercial salve of calendula and eastern white cedar (*Thuja occidentalis*) was also used for skin problems. Another salve (purchased from a local herbalist) contained comfrey (*Symphytum officinalis*) and St. John's wort (*Hypericum perforatum*). Fresh leaves of yellow dock (*Rumex crispus*) are used on nettle stings.

Commercial calendula cream/ointment/gels are used externally for skin problems and burns. Alternatively an external wash was made with 240 ml (1 cup) calendula flowers to 475 ml of water, or a tea was made with 240 ml (1 cup) of calendula flowers to 475 ml of water. It was administered with a syringe (5 to 10 ml per 18 kg dog). Alternatively 0.1 ml of Rescue Remedy (hompeopathic tincture) was given orally.

Ethnoveterinary remedies for a skin problem of unknown cause

This skin problem was said to be one that could be confused with pyoderma (moist eczema), seborrhea, dermatitis, many parasitic or bacterial infections.

A neutered male Husky/Akita dog, 11 and a half years old, 37.7 kg, had sores on various parts of his body, especially on the abdomen, loss of fur and flaking skin. There were accompanying behavioural problems (aggression, apathy) and recurrent head shaking. The dull, dry fur came off in patches. The problem was attributed to allergies to commercial pet foods. A skin reaction started in the groin (small red spots singly or in patches that itched and were inflamed). The dog licked the area constantly, and a secondary bacterial infection developed.

HIS AILMENT WAS TREATED WITH THREE TINCTURES, AN OIL AND A CRÈME THAT WERE MADE AS FOLLOWS.

	Concentration	Tincture 1	Tincture 2	Tincture 3	Oil	Creme
Total mls		125 ml	250 ml	250 ml	n/a	n/a
Arctium lappa roots	1:5/25%	20 ml	40 ml	15 ml	n/a	n/a
Calendula officinalis flowers (harvested	1:5/25%	20 ml	40 ml		125 ml	n/a

by the respondent)

Urtica dioica aerial parts	2:5/25%	20 ml	40 ml	20 ml	n/a	n/a
Taraxacum officinalis radix leaves and roots	1:5/25%	20 ml	40 ml	15 ml	n/a	n/a
Echinacea purpurea roots	1:5/45%	20 ml	40 ml	20 ml	n/a	n/a
Galium aparine aerial parts	1:5/25%	20 ml	40 ml	15 ml	n/a	n/a
Rumex crispus root	2:5/25%	n/a	10 ml	n/a	n/a	n/a
Taraxacum officinalis folia	1:5/25%	n/a	n/a	15 ml	n/a	n/a
Vegetable glycerine	n/a	n/a	n/a	20 ml	n/a	n/a
Stellaria media (manufactured cream)	n/a	n/a	n/a	n/a	n/a	50 g
Plantago lanceolata (purchased leaf tincture)	n/a	n/a	n/a	n/a	n/a	5 ml
Calendula officinalis tincture	1:5/25%	n/a	n/a	n/a	n/a	5 ml
Symphytum officinalis mature leaves (Harvested by respondent)	n/a	n/a	n/a	n/a	250 ml	n/a
Administration	n/a	Evaporate alcohol from 2.5 ml tincture in 15 ml boiling water, wait 10 minutes, mix diluted 2.5 ml twice a day into the food (5 ml per day total ingested).	Evaporate alcohol from 2.5 ml tincture in 15 ml boiling water, wait 10 minutes, mix diluted 2.5 ml twice a day into the food (5 ml per day total ingested).	3.5 ml twice a day mixed into the food	Oil infusions of calendula flowers and comfrey leaves were added to 400 IU Vitamin E. Applied externally.	Applied externally.
Duration of treatment		24 days	50 days	35.7 days	As needed	As needed

At the first consultation the dog was given tincture formula 1, cream, and a Bach flower essence formulation of crabapple (*Malus pumila*), olive (*Olea europeae*), star of Bethlehem (*Ornithogalum umbellatum*), and walnut (*Juglans regia*).

The diet was changed at the first consultation to a raw chicken 60%, oats/barley/millet 20%, and fresh raw vegetables (20%). The following supplements were recommended: vitamin C- 500 mg twice daily; 400 IU vitamin E once daily, 5 ml Cod liver oil every second day; Quercitin- ½ human dose daily; B complex- ½ human dose daily, 5 grams (1 tsp) kelp daily; 5 grams alfalfa daily; 3.5 grams digestive enzymes per meal; 50 mg COQ 10 daily; 20 mg zinc daily; 20 ml flax oil twice daily; Acidophilus- 1/2 human dose.

At the second consultation tincture formula 2 was recommended. An infusion was made with oils and Bach flower essence formulation of: Crabapple, White Chestnut (*Aesculus hippocastanum*), Olive and Rock Rose (*Helianthenum nummularium*).

At the third consultation the herbalist recommended tincture formula 3 and Bach flower essence chicory (*Cichorium intybus*).

Within a week of beginning the new diet and supplements the dog's head shaking stopped and his behavioural problems disappeared. His skin began to clear within two months of the new regime and by three months his skin had completely healed and his fur began to regrow.

Treatment for skin yeast infections

An infusion of fireweed (*Chamerion angustifolium*) is made with 120 ml (½ cup) flowers in 475 ml boiling water (5 ml for every 5 kg bodyweight given twice to three times daily). Long term use was considered safe. A diluted calendula tincture is also used for internally and externally for yeast infections (e.g. *Malassezia pachydermatis*, *Cryptococcus neoformans* varieties *gattii* and *grubii*). Ten drops of tincture are diluted in 30 ml water and given twice daily to small animals (doubled for larger animals). A typical purchased tincture contained 1:5 flowers in 25% alcohol. Long term use is considered safe. Sugar is eliminated from the pet's food.

Treatment for seasonal skin allergies in dogs

Purchased products/decoctions/juices/tinctures of fresh or dried plant tops of stinging nettles (*Urtica dioica*) and chopped burdock root (*Arctium lappa*) are fed daily or every second day to treat skin allergies and itches during seasonal changes (i.e. Winter to Spring), 5 ml daily is fed for five days. The nettles infusion (5 ml (2 tsp) dried leaves in 0.7 litres of water) is kept for 2 days in the fridge; 0.23 litres is fed or 0.11 litres if combined with the burdock tincture. Burdock tincture (1 part fresh chopped burdock root to three parts of a 30% vodka/water solution in a glass container);

Treatment for inhalant atopic dermatitis

A case of inhalant atopic dermatitis was diagnosed by a veterinarian. Specific patient: 8 year old female Dalmation, 29 kgs. Signs were itching and scratching, hay fever, no allergies. The treatment below was tried on 10 dogs and produced good results for three of them, including the Dalmation. Internal treatment: capsules that contained Oregon grape root (*Mahonia aquifolium*), aerial parts nettles (*Urtica dioica*), burdock root (*Arctium lappa*) and licorice root (*Glycyrrhiza glabra*) (50mg for 4.5 kg body weight, given twice daily with food). The treatment is used two weeks on, one week off. Four weeks of treatment were needed for complete resolution of dermatitis/itching. Irregular scratching had been on-going for several years in some of these ten cases.

Supportive therapy:

1. Continued raw, ground rabbit meat as a protein source for a few months for one pet diagnosed as a "hot dog" in Chinese herbal terminology.

2. Commercial Quercenol product containing milk thistle (*Silybum marianum*), vitamin E, proanthocyanins, green tea, zinc, selenium and quercetin.

3. Uncooked bones.

Treatment for allergies in pets

A tea is made from 60 ml (¼ cup) dried mullein leaves (*Verbascum thapsus*) in 0.23 litres of boiling water. The strained tea was given once or twice daily (30 ml) per 4.5kg cat. Cats are given 0.5 capsule of vitamin E or 50 IUs. A 45.5 kg dog is given 30 ml ground flax oil or essential fatty acids or pumpkin, borage or salmon oils. These products are refrigerated for only three days or frozen to avoid rancidity. These oils are put on the food, daily indefinitely as a preventative measure.

4. Discussion

The non-experimental validation of the plants, performed as described in the introductory chapter, is provided in Table 13. A literature review follows.

Zemaphyte, a commercial preparation based on a Chinese formula used in a double-blind placebo-controlled crossover trial of children with atopic eczema, inhibited interleukin (IL)-4-mediated induction of the low-affinity immunoglobulin (Ig)E receptor (CD23) on mononuclear cells (Sheehan et al., 1995; Nagle et al., 2001). The plants tested on 50 dogs with year-round pruritus were *Glycyrrhiza uralensis*, *Paeonia lactiflora* and *Rehmannia glutinosa* and the product produced significant reductions in erythema and surface damage scores with no adverse effects, when administered for 8 weeks. A follow-up study with 120 dogs found that the three –plant product was as good as, or superior to systemic steroid-sparing agents such as antihistamines, pentoxifylline, arofylline, leukotriene inhibitors and misoprostol (Ferguson et al., 2006). Inconclusive results were obtained in an efficacy trial of topical application of capsaicin (0.025%) to treat pruritus in dogs with atopic dermatitis in a double-blinded, placebo-controlled study (Marcella et al., 2002).

Skin problems like atopic dermatitis can have an immunological basis (Lee et al., 2006). T-helper (Th) 2 cytokines are involved at the onset and development of atopic dermatitis, and many patients have peripheral blood eosinophilia and increased serum IgE concentrations. Arctigenin from *Arctium lappa* can modulate immunologic responses (Awale et al., 2006). There is evidentiary support for the anti-inflammatory, anti-infective and vulnerary external applications of *Hypericum perforatum* (O'Hara and Kiefer, 1998; Babenko and Shakhova 2006; Middleton et al., 2000). *Rumex japonicus* can be used for atopic dermatitis (Lee et al., 2006). It contains anthraquinone derivatives, including emodin, chrysophanol and physcion. Linoleic acid is found in (in the seeds of) calendula (*Calendula officinalis*), nettles (*Urtica dioica*), burdock (*Arctium lappa*), plantain (*Plantago major*) and thyme (*Thymus vulgaris*). *Thymus vulgaris* also contains alpha linolenic acid (Duke, 2008). Dietary supplementation of essential fatty acids (linoleic acid, alpha linolenic and gamma linolenic acid) is beneficial for canine atopic dermatitis which may be partially caused by inappropriate eicosanoid synthesis (Saevik et al., 2004). The dietary fatty acid may aid the production of less inflammatory eicosanoids, may inhibit cellular activation and excretion of various cytokines and may contribute to the integrity of the epidermal lipid barrier.

Aesculus hippocastanum increases venous tone, venous flow and lymphatic flow. It also decreases edema formation of lymphatic and inflammatory origin (Mashour et al., 1998). Six triterpene glycosides from the methanol extract of *Calendula officinalis* flowers showed potent inhibitory effects with ID50 values of 0.05-0.32 mg/mouse ear that were comparable to the anti-inflammatory agent indomethacin (Ukiya et al. 2006). Topical *Glycyrrhiza* gel is effective in treating human atopic dermatitis, and has potential as an antiinflammatory treatment for allergic/inflammatory diseases of the skin (Brush et al., 2006). Revitonil (a combination of extracts of *Echinacea* and *Glycyrrhiza*) increased CD69 expression on 30%–50% of T-cells in mice, and stimulated phagocytosis by human granulocytes *in vitro* (Brush et al., 2006).

Aloe vera has anti-fungal and anti-bacterial activity and it decreases vasoconstriction and platelet aggregation by decreasing thromboxane A2 and B2 and prostaglandin F2alpha (Bedi and Shenefelt, 2002). This prevents tissue loss from poor blood supply. It also has pain relieving agents (carboypeptidase, salicylic acid), anti-inflammatory properties (acetylated mannans) and magnesium lactate which acts as an anti-pruritic by inhibiting histidine decarboxylase (histidine to histamine conversion in mast cells).

A mixture of 70% oily extract of *Hypericum* and 30% oily extract of *Calendula* placed on sterile gauzes was tested experimentally on 2 groups of 12 female patients (mean age 33±3 years), who had had caesarean sections during childbirth. The control group was similarly treated for 16 days twice daily with wheat germ oil. The area of the surgical wound at the surface perimeter in the herbal group was reduced by 37.6±9.9% compared to a reduction of 15.83±4.64% in the control group (Lavagna et al., 2001).

The German Commission E monographs on herbal medicines for topical treatment of skin inflammation were aligned with two of the herbal treatments described in this chapter - plantain (*Plantago major*) and fenugreek (*Trigonella foenum-graecum*) (Millikan, 2003). The antimicrobial activity observed in *E. angustifolium* preparations provides a scientific basis for its use in antiseptic and antimycotic remedies to treat eczema, seborrhea, psoriasis and other skin conditions (Batinelli et al., 2001). The Chinese herbal therapy for atopic eczema (Sheehan et al., 1995) continued to show benefits one year after the initial treatment and the herbs produced a strong, dose-dependent, inhibitory effect on CD23 expression in peripheral blood monocytes, not seen in the placebo group (Koo and Desai, 2003). The 14 patients who discontinued the treatment deteriorated. *Chamerion angustifolium* aqueous root extract had activity against *Candida glabrata*, *Candida parapsilosis*, *Cryptococcus neoformans* and *Candida lusitaniae* at low concentrations, and some activity against *Saccharomyces cerivisiae* at 50 mg/l. The active components of the extract are polar compounds found in both aqueous and alcohol extracts (Webster et al., 2008).

It is likely that fenugreek (TRIGONELLA *foenum graecum*), plantain (*Plantago* spp.), mullein (*Verbascum thapsus*), *Aloe vera* and licorice (*Glycyrrhiza uralensis*) are effective in treating skin diseases and merit further study. More research is needed on phytotherapies such as *Chamerion angustifolium* in our study that could be active against the yeasts *Malassezia furfur* and *Malassezia pachydermatis* often found in dogs with atopic dermatitis. Such research has already been conducted with tea tree oil, *Usnea barbata* and *Salvia officinalis* (Weseler et al., 2004; Weckesser et al., 2007).

References

Awale S, Lu J, Kalauni SK, Kurashima Y, Tezuka Y, Kadota S, et al. Identification of arctigenin as an antitumor agent having the ability to eliminate the tolerance of cancer cells to nutrient starvation. *Cancer Res.* 2006; 66:1751 – 1757.

Babenko NA, Shakhova EG. Effects of *Chamomilla recutita* flavonoids on age-related liver sphingolipid turnover in rats. *Exp Gerontol.* 2006; 41:32-9.

Battinelli L, Tita B, Evandri MG, Mazzanti G. Antimicrobial activity of *Chamerion* spp. extracts. *Farmaco.* 2001; 56:345-8.

Bedi MK, Shenefelt PD. Herbal therapy in dermatology. *Arch Dermatol.* 2002; 138:1613.

Bin-Hafeez B, Haque R, Parvez S, Pandey S, Sayeed I, et al. Immunomodulatory effects of fenugreek (*Trigonella foenum graecum* L.) extract in mice. *Int Immunopharmacol.* 2003; 3:257-65.

Bonjar GH. Inhibition of Clotrimazole-resistant *Candida albicans* by plants used in Iranian folkloric medicine. *Fitoterapia* 2004; 75:74-6.

Brush J, Mendenhall E, Guggenheim A, Chan T, Connelly E, et al. The effect of *Echinacea purpurea, Astragalus membranaceus* and *Glycyrrhiza glabra* on CD69 expression and immune cell activation in humans. *Phytother. Res.* 2006; 20: 687–695.

Cho MK, Jang YP, Kim YC, Kim SG. Arctigenin, a phenylpropanoid dibenzylbutyrolactone lignan, inhibits MAP kinases and AP-1 activation via potent MKK inhibition: the role in TNF-alpha inhibition. *Int Immunopharmacol.* 2004; 4:1419-29.

Dal'Belo SE, Gaspar LR, Maia Campos PM. Moisturizing effect of cosmetic formulations containing *Aloe vera* extract in different concentrations assessed by skin bioengineering techniques. *Skin Res Technol.* 2006; 12:241-6.

Di Mambro VM, Fonseca MJ. Assays of physical stability and antioxidant activity of a topical formulation added with different plant extracts. *J Pharm Biomed Anal.* 2005; 37:287-95.

Do Monte FH, dos Santos JG Jr, Russi M, Lanziotti VM, Leal LK, et al. Antinociceptive and anti-inflammatory properties of the hydroalcoholic extract of stems from *Equisetum arvense* L. in mice. *Pharmacol Res.* 2004; 49: 239-43.

Dorhoi A, Dobrean V, Zahan M, Virag P. Modulatory effects of several herbal extracts on avian peripheral blood cell immune responses. *Phytother. Res.* 2006; 20: 352–358.

Duke J A. *Phytochemical and Ethnobotanical Databases*. 2008; USDA-ARS-NGRL, Beltsville Agricultural Research Center, Beltsville, Maryland, USA.

Ferguson EA, Littlewood JD, Carlotti D-N, Grover R, Nuttall T. Management of canine atopic dermatitis using the plant extract PYM00217: a randomized, double-blind, placebo-controlled clinical study. *Vet. Dermatol.* 2006; 17: 236–243.

Filburn CR, Kettenacker R, Griffin DW. Bioavailability of a silybin-phosphatidylcholine complex in dogs. *J Vet Pharmacol Ther.* 2007; 30:132-8.

Fujimura T, Tsukahara K, Moriwaki S, Hotta M, Kitahara T, et al. A horse chestnut extract, which induces contraction forces in fibroblasts, is a potent anti-aging ingredient. *J Cosmet Sci.* 2006; 57:369-76.

Getie M, Gebre-Mariam T, Rietz R, Hohne C, Huschka C, et al. Evaluation of the anti-microbial and anti-inflammatory activities of the medicinal plants *Dodonaea viscosa*, *Rumex nervosus* and *Rumex abyssinicus*. *Fitoterapia* 2003; 74:139-43.

Gülçin I, Küfrevioğlu OI, Oktay M, Büyükokuroğlu ME. Antioxidant, antimicrobial, antiulcer and analgesic activities of nettle (*Urtica dioica* L.). *J Ethnopharmacol.* 2004; 90: 205-15.

Hersch-Martinez P, Leanos-Miranda BE, Solorzano-Santos F. Antibacterial effects of commercial essential oils over locally prevalent pathogenic strains in Mexico. *Fitoterapia* 2005; 76:453-7.

Holetz FB, Pessini GL, Sanches NR, Cortez DA, Nakamura CV, et al. Screening of some plants used in the Brazilian folk medicine for the treatment of infectious diseases. *Mem Inst Oswaldo Cruz* 2002; 97:1027-31.

Iauk L, Costanzo R, Caccamo F, Rapisarda A, Musumeci R, et al. Activity of *Berberis aetnensis* root extracts on Candida strains. *Fitoterapia* 2007; 78:159-61.

Johnson VJ, He Q, Osuchowski MF, Sharma RP. Physiological responses of a natural antioxidant flavonoid mixture, silymarin, in BALB/c mice: III. Silymarin inhibits T-lymphocyte function at low doses but stimulates inflammatory processes at high doses. *Planta Med.* 2003; 69:44-9.

Koo J, Desai R. Traditional Chinese medicine in dermatology. *Dermatol Ther.* 2003; 16:98-105.

Kuiate JR, Bessiere JM, Zollo PH, Kuate SP. Chemical composition and antidermatophytic properties of volatile fractions of hexanic extract from leaves of *Cupressus lusitanica* Mill. from Cameroon. *J Ethnopharmacol.* 2006; 103:160-5.

Lans C, Turner N, Khan T, Brauer G. Ethnoveterinary medicines used to treat endoparasites and stomach problems in pigs and pets in British Columbia, Canada. *Vet. Parasitol* 2007; 148: 325–340.

Lavagna SM, Secci D, Chimenti P, Bonsignore L, Ottaviani A, et al. Efficacy of *Hypericum* and *Calendula* oils in the epithelial reconstruction of surgical wounds in childbirth with caesarean section. *Farmaco.* 2001; 56:451-3.

Lee HS, Kim SK, Han JB, Choi HM, Park JH, et al. Inhibitory effects of *Rumex japonicus* Houtt. on the development of atopic dermatitis-like skin lesions in NC/Nga mice. *Br J Dermatol.* 2006; 155: 33-8.

Luo CN, Lin X, Li WK, Pu F, Wang LW, et al. Effect of berbamine on T-cell mediated immunity and the prevention of rejection on skin transplants in mice. *J Ethnopharmacol.* 1998; 59:211-5.

Marsella R, Nicklin CF, Melloy C. The effects of capsaicin topical therapy in dogs with atopic dermatitis: a randomized, double-blinded, placebo-controlled, cross-over clinical trial. *Vet Dermatol.* 2002; 13:131-9.

Mashour NH, George IL, Frishman WH. Herbal medicine for the treatment of cardiovascular disease. *Arch Intern Med.* 1998; 158: 2225 – 2234.

McQuestion M. Evidence-based skin care management in radiation therapy. *Semin Oncol Nurs.* 2006; 22:163-73.

Mekhfi H, Haouari ME, Legssyer A, Bnouham M, Aziz M, et al. Platelet anti-aggregant property of some Moroccan medicinal plants. *J Ethnopharmacol.* 2004; 94: 317-22.

Middleton E Jr, Kandaswami C, Theoharides TC. The effects of plant flavonoids on mammalian cells: Implications for inflammation, heart disease, and cancer. *Pharmacol Rev*. 2000; 52:673-751.

Millikan LE. Alternative therapy in pruritus. *Dermatol Ther*. 2003; 16:175-80.

Nagle TM, Torres SM, Horne KL, Grover R, Stevens MT. A randomized, double-blind, placebo-controlled trial to investigate the efficacy and safety of a Chinese herbal product (P07P) for the treatment of canine atopic dermatitis. *Vet Dermatol* 2001; 12:265-74.

Patlolla JM, Raju J, Swamy MV, Rao CV. Beta-escin inhibits colonic aberrant crypt foci formation in rats and regulates the cell cycle growth by inducing p21(waf1/cip1) in colon cancer cells. *Mol Cancer Ther*. 2006; 5:1459-66.

Psotova J, Svobodova A, Kolarova H, Walterova D. Photoprotective properties of *Prunella vulgaris* and rosmarinic acid on human keratinocytes. *J Photochem Photobiol B*. 2006; 84:167-74.

Rehman J, Dillow JM, Carter SM, Chou J, Le B, et al. Increased production of antigen-specific immunoglobulins G and M following *in vivo* treatment with the medicinal plants *Echinacea angustifolia* and *Hydrastis canadensis*. *Immunol Lett*. 1999; 68: 391-5.

Saevik BK, Bergvall K, Holm BR, Saijonmaa-Koulumies LE, Hedhammar A, et al. A randomized, controlled study to evaluate the steroid sparing effect of essential fatty acid supplementation in the treatment of canine atopic dermatitis. *Vet Dermatol*. 2004; 15:137-45.

Sancheti G, Goyal PK. Effect of *Rosmarinus officinalis* in modulating 7,12-dimethylbenz(a)anthracene induced skin tumorigenesis in mice. *Phytother Res*. 2006; 20:981-6.

Schempp CM, Windeck T, Hezel S, Simon JC. Topical treatment of atopic dermatitis with St. John's wort cream--a randomized, placebo controlled, double blind half-side comparison. *Phytomedicine* 2003; 10 Suppl 4:31-7.

Schütz K, Carle R, Schieber, A. Taraxacum--a review on its phytochemical and pharmacological profile. *J Ethnopharmacol*. 2006; 107:313-23.

Sheehan MP, Stevens H, Ostlere LS, Atherton DJ, Brostoff J, et al. Follow-up of adult patients with atopic eczema treated with Chinese herbal therapy for 1 year. *Clin Exp Dermatol.* 1995; 20:136-40.

Simou C, Thoday KL, Forsythe PJ, Hill PB. Adherence of *Staphylococcus intermedius* to corneocytes of healthy and atopic dogs: effect of pyoderma, pruritus score, treatment and gender. *Vet Dermatol.* 2005; 16:385-91.

Spelman K, Burns J, Nichols D, Winters N, Ottersberg S, et al. Modulation of cytokine expression by traditional medicines: A review of herbal immunomodulators. *Altern Med Rev.* 2006; 11:128-50.

Štajner D, Popović BM, Boža P. Evaluation of willow herb's (*Chamerion angustofolium* L.) antioxidant and radical scavenging capacities. *Phytother. Res.* 2007; 21: 1242–1245.

Sunila ES, Kuttan G. 2005. Protective effect of *Thuja occidentalis* against radiation-induced toxicity in mice. *Integr Cancer Ther.* 4:322-8.

TAHCC. Alternative Animal Health Care in British Columbia: a manual of traditional practices used by herbalists, veterinarian, farmers and animal caretakers. The Traditional Animal Health Care Collaborative; 2004. Victoria, BC, Canada.

Tanaka Y, Kikuzaki H, Fukuda S, Nakatani, N. Antibacterial compounds of licorice against upper airway respiratory tract pathogens. *J Nutr Sci Vitaminol.* 2001; 47: 270-3.

Turchetti B, Pinelli P, Buzzini P, Romani A, Heimler D, et al. *In vitro* antimycotic activity of some plant extracts towards yeast and yeast-like strains. *Phytother Res.* 2005; 19:44-9.

Turker U, Camper ND. Biological activity of common mullein, a medicinal plant. *J Ethnopharmacol.* 2002; 82:117 – 125.

Turker AU, Usta C. Biological screening of some Turkish medicinal plant extracts for antimicrobial and toxicity activities. *Nat Prod Res.* 2008; 22:136-46.

Uchiyama Y, Tagami J, Kamisuki S, Kasai N, Oshige M, et al. Selective inhibitors of terminal deoxyribo-nucleotidyltransferase (TdT): baicalin and genistin. *Biochim Biophys Acta.* 2005; 1725:298-304.

Ukiya M, Akihisa T, Yasukawa K, Tokuda H, Suzuki T, et al. Anti-Inflammatory, anti-tumor-promoting, and cytotoxic activities of constituents of marigold (*Calendula officinalis*) flowers. *J. Nat. Prod.* 2006; 69: 1692 – 1696.

Wagner H, Jurcic K. Immunological studies of Revitonil, a phytopharmaceutical containing *Echinacea purpurea* and *Glycyrrhiza glabra* root extract. *Phytomedicine*. 2002; 9:390-7.

Webster D, Taschereau P, Belland RJ, Crystal S, Rennie RP. Antifungal activity of medicinal plant extracts; preliminary screening studies. *J Ethnopharmacol.* 2008; 115:140-6.

Weckesser S, Engel K, Simon-Haarhaus B, Wittmer A, Pelz K, et al. Screening of plant extracts for antimicrobial activity against bacteria and yeasts with dermatological relevance. *Phytomedicine.* 2007; 14:508-16.

Wynn SG, Chalmers S. Alternative therapies for pruritic skin disorders. *Clin. Tech. Small. Anim. Pract.* 2002; 17: 37-40.

Yen CH, Dai YS, Yang YH, Wang LC, Lee JH, et al. Linoleic acid metabolite levels and transepidermal water loss in children with atopic dermatitis. *Ann Allergy Asthma Immunol.* 2008; 100:66-73.

Yun SY, Hur YG, Kang MA, Lee J, Ahn C et al. Synergistic immunosuppressive effects of rosmarinic acid and rapamycin *in vitro* and *in vivo. Transplantation* 2003; 75:1758-60.

TABLE 12. ETHNOVETERINARY PLANTS USED FOR PETS IN BRITISH COLUMBIA FOR SKIN PROBLEMS, WOUNDS, SEASONAL ALLERGIES AND INHALANT ATOPIC DERMATITIS

Scientific name	Common name	Plant part used	Ethnoveterinary Use
Aesculus hippocastanum L. (Hippocastanaceae)	horse chestnut	bark, fruit	skin problems
Aloe vera L. (Liliaceae)	Aloe vera	gel	skin regeneration
Arctium lappa L. (Asteraceae)	burdock	roots, rhizomes	unknown skin problem
Calendula officinalis L. (Asteraceae)	calendula	flowers	external & internal treatment, burns, unknown skin problems, yeast infection
Cupressus sempervirens L. var. *dupreziana* (A. Camus) Silba (Cupressaceae)	cypress	needle oil	skin problems
Echinacea purpurea (L.) Moench (Asteraceae)	purple coneflower	roots	unknown skin problem
Chamerion augustifolium L. (Onagraceae)	fireweed	flowers	yeast infection
Equisetum palustre L. (Equisetaceae)	horsetail	aerial parts	abscesses
Galium aparine L. (Rubiaceae)	cleavers	aerial parts	unknown skin problem
Hydrastis canadensis L. (Ranunculaceae)	goldenseal	root	skin problems
Hypericum perforatum L. (Hypericaceae)	St. John's wort	flowers	skin problems
Plantago major L. (Plantaginaceae)	plantain	leaves	unknown skin problem
Rosmarinus officinalis L. (Lamiaceae)	rosemary	aerial parts	skin problems
Rumex crispus L. (Polygonaceae)	yellow dock	leaves	nettle stings, roots for unknown skin problems
Stellaria media (L.) Vill. (Caryophyllaceae)	chickweed	aerial parts	unknown skin problem
Symphytum officinalis L. (Boraginaceae)	comfrey	leaves	unknown skin problem
Taraxacum officinale Weber (Asteraceae)	dandelions	leaves, roots	unknown skin problem
Thuja occidentalis L. (Pinaceae)	Eastern white cedar	twigs	skin problems
Thymus vulgaris L. (Lamiaceae)	thyme	aerial parts	skin problems

Trigonella foenum-graecum L. (Fabaceae)	fenugreek	seeds	skin problems
Urtica dioica L. (Urticaceae)	nettles	aerial parts	unknown skin problem
Arctium lappa L. (Asteraceae)	burdock	root	inhalant atopic dermatitis, seasonal allergies
Berberis aquifolium Pursh./ *Mahonia aquifolium* (Berberidaceae)	Oregon grape	root	inhalant atopic dermatitis
Glycyrrhiza glabra L. (Fabaceae)	licorice	root	inhalant atopic dermatitis
Silybum marianum (L.) Gaertn. (Asteraceae)	Milk thistle	seeds	inhalant atopic dermatitis
Urtica dioica L. (Urticaceae)	nettles	aerial parts	inhalant atopic dermatitis, seasonal allergies
Verbascum thapsus L. (Scrophulariaceae)	mullein	leaves	allergies

Table 13. Non experimental validation of plants used for skin, ear and other problems in pets in British Columbia

Medicinal plant	Validation information	Reference	Validation score
Aesculus hippocastanum	Ethnoveterinary use -skin problems An extract of horse chestnuts (*Aesculus hippocastanum*) can generate contraction forces in fibroblasts. The extract from the seeds of *Aesculus hippocastanum* protects blood vessels, is anti-inflammatory, and has astringent properties causing it to constrict blood vessels. It contains a group of triterpene glycosides (saponins), termed escin (or aescin), which inhibit both elastase and hyaluronidase, and may protect the vessels from degradation by these enzymes. Beta-escin may have anti-inflammatory,	Fujimura et al., 2006; Patiolla et al., 2006	3

	anti-hyaluronidase, and anti-histamine properties.		
Aloe vera / Aloe barbadensis	Ethnoveterinary use - skin regeneration The polysaccharide-rich composition of *Aloe vera* extracts (freeze-dried) was evaluated on skin hydration, after a single and a 1- and 2-week period of application. The extract was applied to the volar forearm of 20 female subjects. After a single application, only formulations supplemented with 0.25% and 0.50% (w/w) of *Aloe vera* extract increased the water content of the stratum corneum, while after the 2-week period application, all formulations containing the extract (0.10%, 0.25% and 0.50%) had the same effect as the vehicle. Freeze-dried *Aloe vera* extract is an effective ingredient for improving skin hydration.	Dal'Belo et al., 2006	4
Arctium lappa	Ethnoveterinary use -case study - unknown skin problem Mixtures of *Glycyrrhiza glabra, Symphytum officinale* and *Arctium majus* root, *Nelumbium speciosum* and soybean showed moderate antioxidant activity and could be used in topical formulations in order to protect skin against damage caused by free radical and reactive oxygen species.	Di Mambro et al., 2005	2
Arctium lappa	Burdock is used for pets with inhalant atopic dermatitis and seasonal allergies *Arctium lappa* has anticandidal activity. Baicalin is known to be an anti-inflammatory or antipyretic agent. Arctigenin is a lignan with antioxidant and anti-inflammatory activities.	Holetz et al., 2002; Uchiyama et al., 2005 ; Cho et al., 2004	2
Berberis	Oregon grape was given to pets with	Iauk et al., 2007;	3

aquifolium / *Mahonia aquifolium*	inhalant atopic dermatitis Berberine's anti-inflammatory action may be due to inhibition of DNA synthesis in activated lymphocytes. Berbamine produced significant supression of the immune functions and prolongation of allograft survival in a mouse skin model of allograft rejection.	Luo et al., 1998	
Calendula officinalis	Ethnoveterinary use - unknown skin problems Surgically-induced standard skin in rats was covered with 5% unguentum containing fractions isolated from the flowers of *Calendula officinalis* in combination with allantoin. It markedly stimulated physiological regeneration and epithelialization. This effect may be due to more intensive metabolism of glycoproteins, nucleoproteins and collagen proteins during the regenerative period in the tissues. Triterpene fatty acid esters isolated from the flower extract show anti-inflammatory and antiedematous activities.	MsQuestion, 2006; Ukiya et al., 2006	4
Cupressus sempervirens	Ethnoveterinary use -skin problems Leaf extracts of *Cupressus sempervirens* were tested against yeast and yeast-like species implicated in human mycoses. It did not have broad antimicrobial activity. *Cupressus lusitanica* fractions showed antidermatophytic activities against *Microsporum audouinii*, *Microsporum langeronii*, *Microsporum canis*, *Trichophyton rubrum* and *Trichophyton tonsurans*.	Turchetti et al., 2005; Kuiate et al., 2006	3
Echinacea purpurea	Ethnoveterinary use - case study unknown skin problems *Echinacea* increased the natural killer (NK) cells and monocytes in both	Brush et al., 2006	3

	bone marrow and spleens of healthy mice compared with controls. Mice with leukemia had more NK cells in their spleens and a longer life than controls. Echinacea's activity is linked to immune cell activation of CD4 and CD8 T cells that have antibacterial activity. *Echinacea spp.* alkamides contribute to its antiinflammatory effects.		
Chamerion augustifolium	Ethnoveterinary use – yeast infection Aqueous extracts of aerial parts of *E. angustifolium* have analgesic and anti-inflammatory activity and reduce the release of prostaglandins. Ethanolic extracts of *E. angustifolium* and alcoholic extracts of *Chamerion* species inhibited the growth of *Staphylococcus aureus, S. albus, Pseudomonas pyocyanea* and *Candida albicans* with MIC values between 81 and 650 µg/ml. The activity of *E. hirsutum* and *E. angustifolium* against *Microsporum canis* was obtained at 10 µg/ml.	Štajner et al., 2007; Battinelli et al., 2001	3
Equisetum palustre	Ethnoveterinary use – abscesses The hydroalchoholic extract of stems of *Equisetum arvense* produced an antinociceptive and anti-inflammatory effects due to beta-sitosterol, campesterol and isofucosterol.	Do Monte et al., 2004	3
Glycyrrhiza glabra	Licorice is used to treat inhalant atopic dermatitis Licorice derived compounds had antiviral and antibacterial activity against upper airway respiratory tract bacteria *Streptococcus pyogenes, Haemophilus influenzae* and *Moraxella catarrhalis*. Licoricidin had the highest activity against all tested microorganisms (MIC of 12.5 microg/mL). Three coumarin derivatives (glycyrol, glycyrin and	Tanaka et al., 2001; Dorhoi et al., 2006	3

	glycycoumarin) had weaker antibacterial activity.		
Hydrastis canadensis	Ethnoveterinary use -skin problems Eight rats were treated with 6.6 g commercially available *Hydrastis canadensis* root extract (concentration 1 g:ml in glycerin solvent) per 1 liter of drinking water. Four control rats received the vehicle glycerin as placebo. A third group of rats was treated with the lower dose of 3.3 g:l of goldenseal extract, which was ineffective. Goldenseal-treated rats had an augmented IgM response during the first 2 weeks of treatment, but failed to show improvement in the IgG response. Herbal treatment did not elevate the maximal immunoglobulin levels, but instead encouraged antibody levels to rise more rapidly.	Rehman et al., 1999	3
Hypericum perforatum	Ethnoveterinary use -skin problems A cream containing *Hypericum* extract standardised to 1.5% hyperforin (verum) was compared to placebo. The study design was a prospective randomised placebo-controlled double-blind monocentric study with twenty one patients suffering from mild to moderate atopic dermatitis. The patients were treated twice daily for four weeks. The hypericum-cream was superior to the vehicle (18 patients completed) in the topical treatment of mild to moderate atopic dermatitis.	Schempp et al., 2003	4
Plantago major	Ethnoveterinary use – unknown skin problems Plantain induces dose dependent proliferation patterns in human lymphocyte cultures. The flavanone glucoside plantagoside is responsible for some of the immunological	Dorhoi et al., 2006; Middleton et al., 2000	3

	activity. Plantagoside is an alpha-mannosidase inhibitor and can potentially restore immune function in immunosuppressed mice.		
Rosmarinus officinalis	Ethnoveterinary use -skin problems *Rosmarinus officinalis* (supercritical carbon dioxide [CO(2)] extracts) was tested for antimicrobial effects on 29 aerobic and anaerobic bacteria and yeasts with dermatological relevance. *Rosmarinus* extract was effective against a panel of microbes including *C. perfringens* and *P. gingivalis* (MIC and MBC<1 mg/ml) and *Candida* yeasts but not against *Klebsiella pneumoniae*. Rosmarinic acid has immuno-suppressive activity and inhibits *in vitro* splenic T-cell proliferation and prolongs skin graft survival *in vivo*. It is useful for the topical treatment of skin disorders like acne vulgaris, tumours and seborrhoic eczema.	Weckesser et al., 2007; Sancheti et al., 2006; Yun et al., 2003	3
Rumex crispus	Ethnoveterinary use - roots for unknown skin problems *Rumex nervosus* leaf extract as well as the extract of the root of *Rumex abyssinicus* have antibacterial activity against *Streptococcus pyogenes* and *Staphylococcus aureus*. *R. abyssinicus* inhibited the synthesis of prostaglandin (PG) E2.	Getie et al., 2003	3
Silybum marianum	Milk thistle is used for inhalant atopic dermatitis in pets *Silybum marianum* demonstrated modulation of multiple cytokines a potential new disease treatment since cytokines are involved in autoimmune conditions and chronic degenerative processes. Silymarin is a mixture of bioactive flavonoids isolated from *Silybum marianum*. *In vitro* studies show that silymarin can inhibit the	Spelman et al., 2006; Johnson et al., 2003; Filburn et al., 2007	3

	production and damage caused by tumor necrosis factor alpha and is a potent antioxidant. *In vivo* parenteral exposure to silymarin results in suppression of T-lymphocyte function at low doses and stimulation of inflammatory processes at higher doses. The activity of silymarin includes inhibition of stellate cell activation, collagen type I synthesis, and resulting fibrogenesis.		
Stellaria media	Ethnoveterinary use – unknown skin problems *Stellaria media* consituents niacin, linoleic acid, mucilage, rutin, zinc and gamma linolenic acid may contribute to its activity against skin problems.	Duke et al., 2008; 50; 3	3
Symphytum officinale	Ethnoveterinary use – unknown skin problems Comfrey has anti-inflammatory activity partially due to rosmarinic acid, a suggested cosmetic ingredient.	Duke et al., 2008; Psotova et al., 2006	3
Taraxacum officinale	Ethnoveterinary use -case study - unknown skin problem *Taraxacum officinale* has shown antiinflammatory activity in many studies.	Schütz et al., 2006	3
Thuja occidentalis	Ethnoveterinary use -skin problems Whole-body exposure of Swiss albino mice to gamma-rays reduced the total white blood cell count to 1900 cells/mm(3) on the third day, which was elevated to 2050 cells/mm(3) when the alcoholic extract of *T occidentalis* (5 mg/dose/animal) was given intraperitoneally. In *T. occidentalis*-treated animals, bone marrow cellularity was increased to nearly normal levels. Alcoholic extract of *T occidentalis* reduced the elevated levels of GPT and alkaline phosphatase in liver and serum after	Sunila and Kuttan, 2005	3

	irradiation. The lipid peroxidation levels were also lowered in the irradiated animals treated with the *Thuja* extract.		
Thymus vulgaris	Ethnoveterinary use -skin problems *Thymus vulgaris* essential oil showed high and broad antibacterial activity against prevalent pathogenic bacteria 189 Gram (-) and 135 Gram (+) strains in Mexico that were isolated from severely infected pediatric patients. *In vitro* anticandidal activity of the methanol extracts of *Thymus vulgaris* (20 mg/ml) was shown against Clotrimazole-resistant *Candida albicans*. *Thymus vulgaris* had a MIC of 0.62 mg/ml.	Hersch-Martinez et al., 2005; Bonjar, 2004	3
Trigonella foenum-graecum	Ethnoveterinary use -skin problems The immunomodulatory activity of aqueous extract of *Trigonella foenum graecum* was evaluated in mice treated with three doses of extract (50, 100 and 250 mg/kg body weight per os) for 10 days. The *T. foenum graecum* showed a stimulatory effect on immune functions in mice. The higher doses increased bone marrow cell counts.	Bin-Hafeez et al., 2003	3
Urtica dioica	Ethnoveterinary use -skin problems, inhalant atopic dermatitis, seasonal allergies *Urtica dioica* leaves had good inhibitory activity against Gram-positive bacteria *Streptococcus pyogenes*, *Staphylococcus aureus* and *Staphylococcus epidermidis* and *E. coli*, but not against the Gram-negative *P. aeruginosa*. Active compounds like flavonoids and caffeic acid derivatives provide the reported anti-inflammatory, antioxidant and analgesic activities. *Urtica dioica* can stimulate human lymphocyte	Turker and Usta, 2008; Gülçin et al., 2004	3

	proliferation. On isolated rat aorta, the aerial part of *Urtica dioica* produces vasoconstriction, while its roots cause vasodilatation. The anti-aggregant activity of *Urtica dioica* is attributed to tannins and flavonoids.		
Verbascum thapsus	*Verbascum thapsus* is used for allergies in pets The aqueous extract has antibacterial activity against *Klebsiella pneumonia*, *Staphylococcus aureus*, *Staphylococcus epidermidis* and *Escherichia coli*. Mucilaginous constituents are responsible for the soothing actions on mucous membranes, and saponins may be responsible for the expectorant actions of mullein.	Turker and Camper, 2002	3

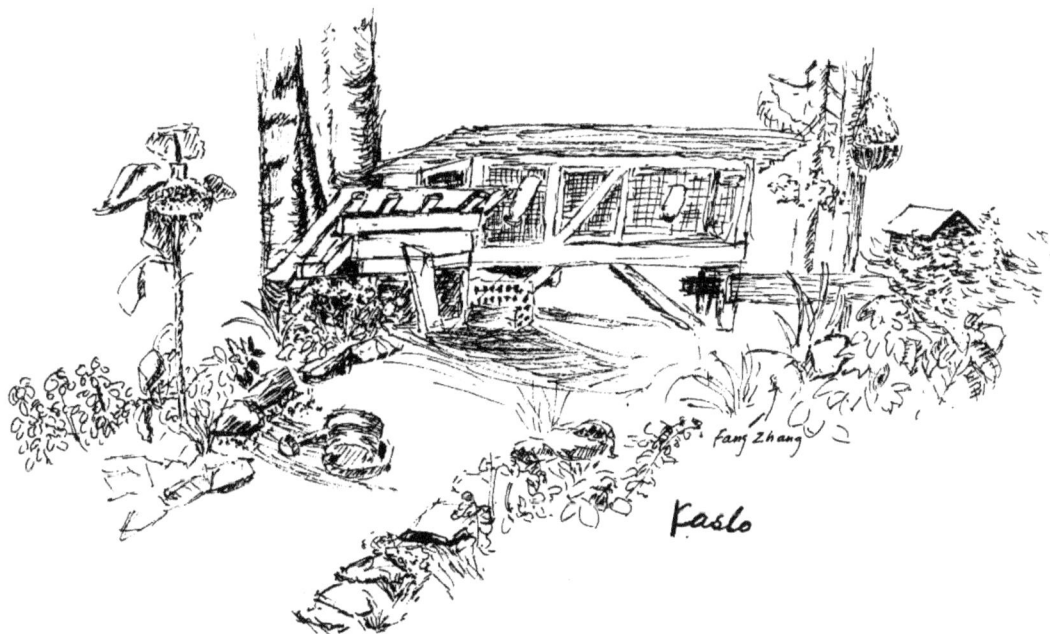

Abstract

Ethnoveterinary data for British Columbia was collected over a six-month period in 2003. This
chapter presents the medicinal plants used for cancer in dogs and cats. Semi-structured
interviews were conducted with 60 participants obtained using a purposive sample.

There are two case studies in the chapter. Dog A was given *Phytolacca decandra*, *Ganoderma
lucidum*, *Lentinula edodes*, *Rumex acetosella* leaf, *Arctium lappa* root, *Ulmus fulva* bark and
Rheum palmatum root. This dog was also given six herbs for lymphatic drainage. Dog B was
given *Frangula purshiana* bark, *Zingiber officinale* root, *Glycyrrhiza glabra* root, *Ulmus fulva* bark,
Althaea officinalis root, *Rheum palmatum* stem, *Rumex crispus* root and *Plantago psyllium* seeds.
Trifolium pratense is used for tumours in the prostate. The following plants are also used to treat
cancer: *Artemisia annua*, *Taraxacum officinale* and *Rumex crispus*. These treatments were said to
prolong the lives of the dogs treated.

Keywords: ethnoveterinary medicine; British Columbia; pets; cancer; tumours; medicinal plants;
mushrooms

1. Introduction

In this chapter we present the medicinal remedies used to treat cancer in pets in British
Columbia, the first chapter of its kind.

A ccording to Balunas and Kinghorn (2005) anticancer agents from plants currently in clinical use can be categorized into four main classes of compounds: vinca (or Catharanthus) alkaloids, epipodophyllotoxins, taxanes, and camptothecins. Vinblastine and vincristine, prescribed for the last four decades, were isolated from *Catharanthus roseus* (L.) G. Don (Apocynaceae) (formerly *Vinca rosea* L.). These vinca alkaloids and several of their semi-synthetic derivatives block mitosis with metaphase arrest by binding specifically to tubulin resulting in its depolymerization. The epipodophyllotoxins bind tubulin, causing breaks in the DNA strand during the G2 phase of the cell cycle by irreversibly inhibiting DNA topoisomerase II. Paclitaxel was originally identified from Pacific yew (*Taxus brevifolia* Nutt. Taxaceae) and has been prescribed in North America since the 1990s. This compound can now be synthesized from base molecules in other *Taxus* spp. The taxanes, including paclitaxel and derivatives, act by binding tubulin without allowing depolymerization or interfering with tubulin assembly. Camptothecin was isolated from *Camptotheca acuminata* Decne. (Nyssaceae) but originally showed unacceptable myelosuppression (Balunas and Kinghorn, 2005). Interest in camptothecin was revived when it was found to act by selective inhibition of topoisomerase I, involved in cleavage and reassembly of DNA. The taxanes and the camptothecins alone accounted for about one-third of the global anticancer market, or more than 2.75 billion dollars in 2002 alone. Podophyllotoxin is a lignan that was isolated from the resin of *Podophyllum peltatum* L. (Berberidaceae), safer derivatives have since been maed, the first being etoposide.

Many commonly used herbs have cancer-preventive properties; several of these herbs are dealt with in this chapter. They include members of the Lamiaceae family (mint, sage, rosemary and thyme); spices of the Zingiberaceae family (turmeric and ginger (*Zingiber officinale*)); licorice root (Fabaceae) and herbs in the Apiaceae family (celery, dill and parsley) (Craig, 1999). These plants typically contain phytosterols, triterpenes, flavonoids, saponins, and carotenoids, which are cancer chemoprotective (Craig, 1999). Some also contain phenolic compounds (e.g. phenolic acids, flavonoids, quinones, coumarins, lignans, stilbenes, tannins), with significant antioxidant activity (Cai et al., 2004).

Many dogs and cats with cancer are older animals. Cyclooxygenase (COX)-2 is an inducible enzyme linked to tumor growth and angiogenesis. COX-2 is expressed in mammary tissues during tumorigenesis and its expression is associated with a poorer prognosis in bitches and queens ($p=0.03$ in dogs and $p=0.002$ in cats) with invasive mammary tumours. COX-2 overexpression in queens was significantly correlated to estrogen receptor (ER) negative status (Millanta et al., 2006; Langsenlehner et al., 2007). COX-2 immunoreactivity was not seen in healthy tissues, but it was detected in 96% of feline and 100% of canine invasive carcinomas (Millanta et al., 2006). Primary lung tumors are less common than metastatic lung lesions in dogs and cats. Adenocarcinomas account for 70% to 80% of primary pulmonary neoplasia in dogs and cats; less common carcinomas include squamous cell carcinomas and adenosquamous carcinomas (Langlais et al., 2006). Metastasis of primary lung tumors in dogs and cats can occur in other areas of the body.

2. Materials and methods

Already described in the introductory chapter.

3. Results

We document two case studies of specific dogs being treated for cancer followed by general treatments used for cancer as identified by our respondents (Table 14). The cancers treated in the case studies were mast cell tumours (legs) and tumours outside the liver and pancreas.

3.1 Treatments used for cancer in pets in British Columbia

Bone cancer in one dog was diagnosed by a veterinarian. The dog was given sweet/annual wormwood (*Artemisia annua*) (200 to 800 mg per day for a 68 to 82 kg animal for six to twelve months, then reduced slowly). The dosage was altered according to the quality of the Artemisia extract.

A 1:1 tincture of red clover (*Trifolium pratense*) in vodka was given to treat tumours. The dose used was 10 drops per 15 lbs bodyweight twice a day for acute cases of cancer. For blood cancer a dog was given 5 drops. The tincture was sprinkled on the food once a week during the winter.

Another treatment used was a tincture of dandelions (*Taraxacum officinale*) in vodka and given in the lip as a supportive treatment (3 – 5 drops per 15 lbs bodyweight). This tincture was used with conventional veterinary treatment (radiation and chemotherapy). Dandelion tea cannot be substituted.

Yellow dock (*Rumex crispus*) (tincture not tea) was used for six months once a day as a treatment for tumours outside the liver and pancreas. Flowers of red clover (*Trifolium pratense*) were used to fight tumour growth in prostate cases. Large dogs are given up to 160 mg/day. Red clover is not used for animals about to have surgery. These treatments were said to prolong the lives of the animals.

3.2 Case study of the treatment for a dog with cancer

All of the treatments below are part of one case study. The 119 lb dog had already been   with diagnosed with cancer (mast cell tumours on the legs) by a veterinarian and was not expected to live. After the treatments, blood work showed less cancer cells. The dog eventually did die of cancer but lived for 2.5 years longer than originally predicted. The products used on this dog and listed below are all human products.

A poultice for the tumours was made with ½ tsp of poke root (*Phytolacca decandra*). A paste was made based on the size of the treated area. It was wrapped with plastic and then bandaged. A tincture of reishi (*Ganoderma lucidum*) and shiitake (*Lentinula edodes*) mushrooms was diluted to the appropriate strength for the pet (40 drops three times a day). After four months the mushroom tincture was reduced to half and the reduced dose was continued for the rest of two years to the end of the patient's life.

A purchased product (Essiac, a well-known herbal remedy used for cancer) containing the following ingredients was administered orally: leaf of sheep sorrel (*Rumex acetosella*), burdock root (*Arctium lappa*), inner bark powder of slippery elm (*Ulmus fulva*) and root of turkey rhubarb (*Rheum palmatum*) (bowel mover). The major product ingredient in the product was sheep sorrel (½ to 2/3 of the weight), then burdock. This product was used three times a day. After four months the dose (of the sheep sorrel combination) was reduced by half and this reduced dose was given for two years to the end of the pet's life.

To drain the lymphatic system of the dog, a purchased tincture was administered internally for three months (40 drops three times a day for a 119 lb animal). It was composed of Oregon grape (*Berberis aquifolium/Mahonia aquifolium*), marshmallow (*Althaea officinalis*), blue flag (*Iris versicolor*), mullein (*Verbascum thapsus*) and root of stillingia (*Stillingia sylvatica*). It is recommended for mast cell tumours external and internal around the organs. Then the dog was given root capsules of dandelions (250 mg) once a day and the Oregon grape combination was discontinued. The sheep sorrel combination treatment was continued. Additionally slippery elm (*Ulmus fulva*) was given orally.

3.3 Plants used to detoxify or purify the blood

Herbalists treating cancer also use herbs for detoxification. A multi-plant decoction used for detoxification includes dandelion root (*Taraxacum officinale*), cleavers (*Galium aparine*) plant, yellow dock root (*Rumex crispus*), yucca root (*Yucca schidigera*) and burdock root (*Arctium lappa*). A decoction is made using l-2 tsp of each in 0.9 litres of water, this is then brought to a boil (dose given is 0.0049 l of tea per 45 kg/ dog given three times a day). If a commercial tincture is available with this combination of herbs, 2 to 5 drops of it (per 11 kg patient bodyweight) is given three times a day.

A single-plant burdock tincture is also used for detoxification. This is made with 1 part fresh chopped burdock root to three parts of a 30% vodka/water solution. Alternatively a burdock decoction is made with 1 tsp of thinly-sliced, fresh or dried burdock root in 0.2 litres water. The decoction is put in the food (0.227 litres) or 0.11 litres if it is combined with nettles.

Yellow dock (*Rumex crispus*) dried shredded or dried chopped root is used as a blood and liver purifier (a 1:1 tincture of root extract and vodka). The pet is given 5 drops per 11.33 kg patient bodyweight twice a day with the morning and evening meal. For acute cases it is used once daily for a month. A decoction made with 1 tsp roots of yellow dock (*Rumex crispus*) in addition to 1 tsp roots of burdock (*Arctium lappa*). This Is put in the food – 0.056 litres for every 22.7 kg bodyweight.

Also used is an infusion of celery (*Apium graveolens*) seeds and stalks (0.227 litres boiling water with 1-2 tsp of freshly crushed seeds per 11.33 kg patient bodyweight).

Borage leaf tea (*Borago officinalis*) is another alternative (0.227 litres boiling water to 2 tsp dried leaves). A combination tea is also made with 2 tsp borage and 1 tsp each of leaves of dandelions (*Taraxacum officinale*) and nettles (*Urtica dioica*) in 0.455 litres boiling water (1 tsp of either tea per 11.33 kg patient bodyweight). Borage is used for only two to three days then the treatment is discontinued since the leaves are said to contain pyrrolizidine alkaloids.

A tincture made with the aerial parts of cleavers (*Galium aparine*) is another plant-based treatment (1/2–1 tsp tincture three times per day). A tea can be made by steeping 2–3 tsp aerial parts in 0.227 litres boiling water. This tea is given at 0.227 litres per day per 18 kg patient bodyweight. Also used for detoxification purposes is lavender flower tea (*Lavandula officinalis*) (5 ml (1 tsp) of dried flowers is steeped in 0.227 litres of boiling water, 0.0568 L daily for a 27 kg dog).

A white willow decoction is also used as a treatment (2 ml (1/2 tsp) of dried willow (*Salix alba*) bark soaked in 0.454 litres of cold water for 10 to 14 hours, then brought to a boil). The dose used is 15 ml (1 tbsp) daily for a 22.7 kg dog. Yarrow tea is another alternative. This is made by steeping 80 ml (1/3 cup) flowers of yarrow (*Achillea millefolium*) in 0.454 litres of boiling water for 15 - 20 minutes (0.0568 litres are given daily per 22.7 kg bodyweight).

A nettles infusion is also used for detoxification. This is made by adding 10 ml (2 tsp) dried leaves of nettles (*Urtica dioica*) to 0.568 litres of water; 0.227 litres of the strained warm or cold infusion is added to the food for an 38.5 kg dog or 0.11 litres if combined with the burdock (*Arctium lappa*) preparation.

Pets are given a 1:1 full strength vodka tincture made with chickweed aerial parts or whole plant (*Stellaria media*) (1 to 2 drops of tincture daily). Alternatively a tea is made with 2 tsp aerial parts in 0.227 litres of boiling water (1 tbsp tea daily per 9 – 13.6 kg patient bodyweight). Pets are given flowers of red clover (*Trifolium pratense)* added to the diet two times a week as a preventative or as a 'blood purifier' (1 – 1.5 tsp every three days for a 38.55 to 45.4 kg dog).

4. Discussion and Conclusion

The non-experimental validation of the plants is presented in Table 15. Several of the plants identified above have been tested against cancer cell lines.

One of the purchased products used for pets seems to be based on Rene Cassie's "Essiac Formula" which is reported to be: 6 1/2 cups burdock root – cut (*Arctium lappa*), 16 oz. sheep sorrel herb – powdered (*Rumex acetosella*), 1 oz. turkey rhubarb root – powdered (*Rheum palmatum*), 4 oz. Slippery elm bark – powdered (*Ulmus fulva*). Clinical trials on this formula have just begun (Zick et al., 2006; Seely et al., 2007).

Lentinan from shiitake mushrooms (*Lentinus edodes*), has antitumor and immune stimulant activity; it was active against lung carcinoma and 2 human melanomas (Craig, 1999).

A review of Chinese medicinal plants used for their reputed anticancer activity or anticarcinogenic and antimutagenic effects found that the commonly found active constituents in these plants include terpenes (sesquiterpenes, diterpenes, triterpenes), alkaloids, lignans, coumarins, tannins, quinones, flavonoids, stilbenes, curcuminoids and polysaccharides; many with antioxidant activity (Cai et al., 2004; Lin and Harnly, 2008 Kardosová et al., 2003). Phenolic acids (chlorogenic acid) and lignans (arctigenin, arctiin) are some of the active compounds found in the fruit of burdock

(*Arctium lappa*); hydroxycinnamoylquinic acids and a fructofuranan are found in the root. Flavones (luteolin, luteolin-7- glucoside), flavonols (kaempferol, quercetin, rutin) and coumarins (coumarin, 6,7-dimethoxy-coumarin) are the major phenolic compounds in Artemisia (*Artemisia annua*). Ginger rhizome (*Zingiber officinale* Rosc.) contains phenolic volatile oils (gingerol analogues: gingerols, shogaol).

Plants cited by Cai et al. (2004), that are closely related to those used in this research include: *Glycyrrhiza uralensis* Fisch. - the root contains flavanones (dihydroflavones: liquiritin, liquirigenin) and licopyranocoumarins. *Plantago asiatica* L. contains flavones (plantaginin); *Crataegus pinnatifida* Bge. - fruit contains flavonoids (epicatechin, quercetin, vitexin, quercitrin) and phenolic acids (chlorogenic acid); *Rheum officinale* Baill.- roots contain anthraquinones (emodin, chrysophanol, rhein, physcion and their glycosides), phenolic acids (gallic acid) and hydrolyzable tannins; and *Taraxacum mongolicum* Hand.–Mazz.- whole plant contains flavonols (rutin). Aqueous extracts of *Rheum palmatum* roots and rhizomes and *Artemisia argyi* leaf showed antiproliferative activity against cancer cell lines (Shoemaker et al., 2005).

Several phytochemicals, including some in the treatments documented, inhibit tumor formation by stimulating the protective phase II enzyme, glutathione transferase; this enzyme helps to form compounds with reduced toxicity that are more water-soluble, that can be excreted easily. Examples of phytochemicals that stimulate glutathione transferase activity include phthalides, found in umbelliferous herbs; sulfides, found in curcumin in turmeric and ginger; and commonly found terpenoids (limonene, geraniol, menthol, and carvone) (Craig, 1999).

Triterpenoid acids, such as oleanolic and ursolic acid (a pentacyclic triterpenoid), are found in lavender (*Lavandula latifolia*), and are associated with weak anti-inflammatory and anti-tumor activities (Cragg and Newman, 2005). Ursolic acid can arrest the Hep G2 cell cycle at G0/G1 phase by inhibiting DNA replication and increasing p21/WAF1 expression. Other studies have shown that ursolic acid can induce apoptosis through calcium-dependent and activation sphingomyelinase (Hsu et al., 2004).

Luteolin is a flavonoid found in some ethnoveterinary remedies described in this study (Table 16). Its anticancer properties include induction of cancer cell apoptosis, cell cycle arrest, inhibition of cancer cell proliferation, and antiangiogenesis activity (Shi et al., 2005).

Stillingia sylvatica, *Althaea officinalis* and *Iris versicolor* are poorly studied, however the other plants discussed in this chapter have moderate to high levels of validity in the treatment of cancer. Many of the studies are very recent and on-going therefore the assessment of validity is based on few studies.

The antitumour activity of medicinal plants is achieved via a number of mechanisms, including stimulation of the immune system, or antiprotease-antioxidant activity (Mantle et al., 2000). Furthermore various bioactive constituents can act as cancer-preventing agents by inhibiting the activation of procarcinogens, stopping carcinogens from interacting with critical target sites, or hindering the progression of carcinogenesis (Tatman and Mo, 2002; Duke, 1990). Examples include ginger (*Zingiber officinale*) with 13,500 ppm of the isoprenoid citral that has an IC50 of 30 ± 10 µmol/l against the B16 melanoma cell line. Ginger also contains geraniol (345 ppm) with an IC50 of 139 ± 27 µmol/l against the B16 melanoma cell line (Tatman and Mo, 2002; Duke, 1990). *Lavandula* X *intermedia* and *Lavandula latifolia* also contain small amounts of geraniol. Celery seed (*Apium graveolens*) has 1ppm of perillaldehyde with an IC50 of 120 ±17 µmol/l against the B16 melanoma cell line.

Another role for herbal remedies may be as immune boosters. *Lentinula edodes* and *Ganoderma lucidum* fall into this role. Studies have shown that cellular immunodeficiency is associated with human cancer. Cancer chemotherapy, particularly with cyclophosphamide, causes a decline in the number of T cells in peripheral blood (Kormosh et al., 2006).

References

Adams, J.DJr., Garcia, C. 2006. Women's health among the Chumash. eCAM 3, 125–131.

Adolf, W., Hecker, E. 1980. New irritant diterpene-esters from roots of *Stillingia sylvatica* L. (Euphorbiaceae). Tetrahedron Lett 21, 2887-2890.

Aksu MG, Bozcuk HS, Korcum AF. 2008. Effect of complementary and alternative medicine during radiotherapy on radiation toxicity. Support Care Cancer 16(4):415-9.

Al-Hindawi, M.K., Al-Deen, I.H., Nabi, M.H., Ismail, M.A. 1989. Anti-inflammatory activity of some Iraqi plants using intact rats. J Ethnopharmacol. 26,163-8.

Anon, 2008. Perillyl Alcohol. http://www.mskcc.org/mskcc/html/69329.cfm

Amirghofran, Z., Bahmani, M., Azadmehr, A., Javidnia, K. 2006. Anticancer effects of various Iranian native medicinal plants on human tumor cell lines. Neoplasma. 53, 428-33.

Awale, S., Lu, J., Kalauni, S.K., Kurashima, Y., Tezuka, Y., Kadota, S., Esumi, H. 2006. Identification of arctigenin as an antitumor agent having the ability to eliminate the tolerance of cancer cells to nutrient starvation. Cancer Res 66, 1751 – 1757.

Balunas, M.J., Kinghorn, A.D. Drug discovery from medicinal plants. Life Sciences 78: 431 – 441.

Blumenthal, M., Goldberg, A., Brinckmann, J, editors. 2000. Herbal Medicine: Expanded Commission E Monographs. Austin, TX: American Botanical Council; Boston: Integrative Medicine Communications.

Cai, Y., Luo, Q., Sun, M., Corke, H. 2004. Antioxidant activity and phenolic compounds of 112 traditional Chinese medicinal plants associated with anticancer. Life Sciences 74, 2157–2184.

Celik I, Tuluce Y. 2007. Elevation protective role of Camellia sinensis and Urtica dioica infusion against trichloroacetic acid-exposed in rats. Phytother Res. 21(11):1039-44.

Chadwick, L.R., Pauli, G.F., Farnsworth, N.R. 2006. The pharmacognosy of *Humulus lupulus* L. (hops) with an emphasis on estrogenic properties. Phytomedicine 13, 119–131.

Cragg, G.M., Newman, D.J. 2005. Plants as a source of anti-cancer agents. Journal of Ethnopharmacology 100, 72–79.

Craig, W.J. 1999. Health-promoting properties of common herbs. Am J Clin Nutr. 70(suppl), 491S–9S.

Durak I, Biri H, Devrim E, Sözen S, Avci A. 2004. Aqueous extract of Urtica dioica makes significant inhibition on adenosine deaminase activity in prostate tissue from patients with prostate cancer. Cancer Biol Ther. 3(9):855-7.

D'Cruz, O.J., Waurzyniak, B., Uckun, F.M. 2004. Mucosal toxicity studies of a gel formulation of native pokeweed antiviral protein. Toxicologic Pathology 32, 212-21.

Duke, J.A. 1990. Promising phytomedicinals. In: J. Janick and J.E. Simon (eds.), Advances in new crops. Timber Press, Portland, OR. p. 491-498.

Elmastas, M., Lokman Ozturk, L., Gokce, I., Erenler, R., Aboul - Enein, H. 2004. Determination of antioxidant activity of marshmallow flower (*Althaea officinalis* L.) Analytical Letters 37, 1859 – 1869.

El-Shemy, H.A., Aboul-Enein, A.M., Aboul-Enein, K.M., Fujita, K. 2007. Willow leaves' extracts contain anti-tumor agents effective against three cell types. PLoS ONE 2(1).

Fine, R.L., Patel, J., Chabner, B.A. 1988. Phorbol esters induce multidrug resistance in human breast cancer cells. Proc Natl Acad Sci U S A., 85, 582-6.

Gu, Y.H., Belury, M.A. 2005. Selective induction of apoptosis in murine skin carcinoma cells (CH72) by an ethanol extract of *Lentinula edodes*. Cancer Lett. 220, 21-8.

Gülçin, I., Küfrevioğlu, O.I., Oktay, M., Büyükokuroğlu, M.E. 2004. Antioxidant, antimicrobial, antiulcer and analgesic activities of nettle (*Urtica dioica* L.). J Ethnopharmacol. 90, 205-15.

Habs, M. 2004. Prospective, comparative cohort studies and their contribution to the benefit assessments of therapeutic options: Heart failure treatment with and without hawthorn special extract WS 1442. Forsch Komplementärmed Klass Naturheilkd 11(suppl 1), 36-39.

Hostanska K, Jürgenliemk G, Abel G, Nahrstedt A, Saller R. 2007. Willow bark extract (BNO1455) and its fractions suppress growth and induce apoptosis in human colon and lung cancer cells. Cancer Detect Prev. 31(2):129-39.

Hsu, Y.-L., Kuo, P.-L., Lin, C-C. 2004. Proliferative inhibition, cell-cycle dysregulation, and induction of apoptosis by ursolic acid in human non-small cell lung cancer A549 cells. Life Sciences 75, 2303–2316.

Iauk, L., Costanzo, R., Caccamo, F., Rapisarda, A., Musumeci, R., Milazzo, I., Blandino, G. 2006. Activity of *Berberis aetnensis* root extracts on Candida strains. Fitoterapia. 78(2):159-61.

Jayalakshmi, R., Niranjali, D. S. 2004. Cardioprotective effect of tincture of Crataegus on isoproterenol-induced myocardial infarction in rats. Journal of Pharmacy and Pharmacology 56(7), 921-6.

Jellinek, N., Maloney, M. 2005. Escharotic and other botanical agents for the treatment of skin cancer: A review. J Am Acad Dermatol 53, 487-95.

Kao ES, Wang CJ, Lin WL, Chu CY, Tseng TH. 2007. Effects of polyphenols derived from fruit of *Crataegus pinnatifida* on cell transformation, dermal edema and skin tumor formation by phorbol ester application. Food Chem Toxicol. 45(10):1795-804.

Kang, Chan-S., Chang, M.L., Choi, H., Lee, J.H., Oh, J.S., Kwak, J.H., Zee, O.P. 2006. Evaluation of oriental medicinal herbs for estrogenic and antiproliferative activities. Phytother. Res. 20, 1017–1019.

Kardosová A, Ebringerová A, Alföldi J, Nosál'ová G, Franová S, Hríbalová V. 2003. A biologically active fructan from the roots of *Arctium lappa* L., var. Herkules. Int J Biol Macromol. 33(1-3):135-40.

Kormosh, N., Laktionov, K., Antoshechkina, M. 2006. Effect of a combination of extract from several plants on cell-mediated and humoral immunity of patients with advanced ovarian cancer. Phytother. Res. 20, 424–425.

Kwok, Y., Ng, K.F., Li, C.C., Lam, C.C., Man, R.Y. 2005. A prospective, randomized, double-blind, placebo-controlled study of the platelet and global hemostatic effects of *Ganoderma lucidum* (Ling-Zhi) in healthy volunteers. Anesth Analg. 101,423-6.

Lai, H., Singh, N.P. 2006. Oral artemisinin prevents and delays the development of 7,12-dimethylbenz[a]anthracene (DMBA)-induced breast cancer in the rat. Cancer Lett. 231,43-8.

Langlais, L.M., Gibson, J., Taylor, J.A., Caswell, J.L. 2006. Pulmonary adenocarcinoma with metastasis to skeletal muscle in a cat. Can Vet J. 47, 1122-3.

Langsenlehner, U., Gerger, A., Weitzer, W., Krippl, P. 2007. COX-2 expression in canine and feline invasive mammary carcinomas: correlation with clinicopathological features and prognostic for molecular markers. Breast Cancer Res Treat. 101, 247.

Lans, C., Turner, N., Brauer, G., Lourenco, G., Georges, K. 2006. Ethnoveterinary medicines used for horses in Trinidad and in British Columbia, Canada. Journal of Ethnobology and Ethnomedicine 2006; 2,31.

Lebedeva IV, Su ZZ, Vozhilla N, Chatman L, Sarkar D, Dent P, Athar M, Fisher PB. 2008. Mechanism of in vitro pancreatic cancer cell growth inhibition by melanoma differentiation-associated gene-7/interleukin-24 and perillyl alcohol. Cancer Res. 68(18):7439-47.

Lin, Liang-Tzung, Liu, Li-Teh, Chiang, Lien-Chai, Lin, Chun-Ching. 2002. *In vitro* anti-hepatoma activity of fifteen natural medicines from Canada. Phytother. Res. 16, 440–444.

Lin LZ, Harnly JM. 2008. Identification of hydroxycinnamoylquinic acids of arnica flowers and burdock roots using a standardized LC-DAD-ESI/MS profiling method. J Agric Food Chem. 56(21):10105-14.

Luo, C.N., Lin, X., Li, W.K., Pu, F., Wang, L.W., Xie, S.S., Xiao, P.G. 1998. Effect of berbamine on T-cell mediated immunity and the prevention of rejection on skin transplants in mice. J Ethnopharmacol. 59,211-5.

Mantle, D., Lennard, T.W., Pickering, A.T. 2000. Therapeutic applications of medicinal plants in the treatment of breast cancer: a review of their pharmacology, efficacy and tolerability. Adverse Drug React Toxicol Rev. 19, 223-40.

Matos JM, Schmidt CM, Thomas HJ, Cummings OW, Wiebke EA, Madura JA, Patrick LJ Sr, Crowell PL. 2008. A pilot study of perillyl alcohol in pancreatic cancer. J Surg Res. 147(2):194-9.

Mavi, A., Terzi, Z., Ozgen, U., Yildirim, A., Coskun, M. 2004. Antioxidant properties of some medicinal plants: *Prangos ferulacea* (Apiaceae), *Sedum sempervivoides* (Crassulaceae), *Malva neglecta* (Malvaceae), *Cruciata taurica* (Rubiaceae), *Rosa pimpinellifolia* (Rosaceae), *Galium verum* subsp. verum (Rubiaceae), *Urtica dioica* (Urticaceae). Biol Pharm Bull. 27, 702-5.

Millanta, F., Citi, S., Della Santa D., Porciani, M., Poli, A. 2006. COX-2 expression in canine and feline invasive mammary carcinomas: correlation with clinicopathological features and prognostic molecular markers. Breast Cancer Res Treat. 2006 98, 115-20.

Min BS, Kim YH, Lee SM, Jung HJ, Lee JS, Na MK, Lee CO, Lee JP, Bae K. 2000. Cytotoxic triterpenes from *Crataegus pinnatifida*. Arch Pharm Res. 23(2):155-8.

Olas, B., Wachowicz, B., Stochmal, A., Oleszek, W. 2005. Inhibition of blood platelet adhesion and secretion by different phenolics from *Yucca schidigera* Roezl. bark. Nutrition 21,199-206.

Park, E., J., Pezzuto, J.M. 2002. Botanicals in cancer chemoprevention. Cancer and Metastasis Reviews 21, 231–255.

Rodríguez-Cabezas ME, Gálvez J, Lorente MD, Concha A, Camuesco D, Azzouz S, Osuna A, Redondo L, Zarzuelo A. 2002. Dietary fiber down-regulates colonic tumor necrosis factor alpha and nitric oxide production in trinitrobenzenesulfonic acid-induced colitic rats. J Nutr. 132(11):3263-71.

Seely D, Kennedy DA, Myers SP, Cheras PA, Lin D, Li R, Cattley T, Brent PA, Mills E, Leonard BJ. 2007. *In vitro* analysis of the herbal compound Essiac. Anticancer Res. 27(6B): 3875-82.

Shia, G., Shaw, D., Dargan, P.I. 2004. Assessing health risks of complementary alternative medicines in cancer patients. British Journal of Cancer 91, 995–996.

Shidoji, Y., Ogawa, H., 2004. Natural occurrence of cancer-preventive geranylgeranoic acid in medicinal herbs. Journal of Lipid Research 45, 1092 – 1103.

Shi, R-X., Ong C-N., Shen H-M. 2005. Protein kinase C inhibition and X-linked inhibitor of apoptosis protein degradation contribute to the sensitization effect of luteolin on tumor necrosis factor–related apoptosis- inducing ligand–induced apoptosis in cancer cells. Cancer Res 65, 7815 – 7823.

Shoemaker, M., Hamilton, B., Dairkee, S.H., Cohen, I., Campbell, M.J. 2005. *In vitro* anticancer activity of twelve Chinese medicinal herbs. Phytother. Res. 19, 649–651.

Singh, N.P., Lai, H. 2001. Selective toxicity of dihydroartemisinin and holotransferrin toward human breast cancer cells. Life Sciences 70, 49-56.

Stoggl, W.M., Huck, C.W., Bonn, G.K. 2004. Structural elucidation of catechin and epicatechin in sorrel leaf extracts using liquid-chromatography coupled to diode array-, fluorescence-, and mass spectrometric detection. J Sep Sci. 27, 524-8.

Tai, J., Cheung, S. 2005. *In vitro* culture studies of FlorEssence on human tumor cell lines. Phytother Res. 19, 107-12.

Tatman, D., Mo, H. 2002. Volatile isoprenoid constituents of fruits, vegetables and herbs cumulatively suppress the proliferation of murine B16 melanoma and human HL-60 leukemia cells. Cancer Lett. 175, 129-39.

Yang, W.H., Wieczorck, M., Allen, M.C., Nett, T.M. 2003. Cytotoxic activity of gonadotropin-releasing hormone (GnRH)-pokeweed antiviral protein conjugates in cell lines expressing GnRH receptors. Endocrinology. 144, 1456-63.

Vermani, K., Garg, S. 2002. Herbal medicines for sexually transmitted diseases and AIDS. Journal of Ethnopharmacology 80, 49-66.

Wagner, H., Jurcic, K. 2002. Immunological studies of Revitonil, a phytopharmaceutical containing *Echinacea purpurea* and *Glycyrrhiza glabra* root extract. Phytomedicine 2002, 9,390-7.

Wynn, S.G., Marsden, S.A. 2003. Manual of natural veterinary medicine: Science and tradition. Mosby: St Louis.

Zick, S.M., Sen, A., Feng, Y., Green, J., Olatunde, S., Boon, H. 2006. Trial of Essiac to ascertain its effect in women with breast cancer (TEA-BC). J Altern Complement Med. 12, 971-80.

TABLE 14. ETHNOVETERINARY TREATMENTS FOR PETS WITH CANCER IN BRITISH COLUMBIA

Scientific name (plant family)	Common name	Plant part used	Use
Achillea millefolium L. (Asteraceae)	yarrow	flowers	detoxification
Althaea officinalis L. (Malvaceae)	marshmallow	root	Dog A cancer lymphatic drainage, Dog B cancer
Apium graveolens L. (Apiaceae)	celery	seeds, stalks	detoxification
Arctium lappa L. (Asteraceae)	burdock	root	Dog A cancer, detoxification
Artemisia sp. (Asteraceae)	sweet wormwood	leaves	Cancer
Berberis aquifolium Pursh./ *Mahonia aquifolium* (Berberidaceae)	Oregon grape	root	Dog A cancer lymphatic drainage
Borago officinalis L. (Boraginaceae)	borage	leaves	detoxification
Crataegus oxycantha (Rosaceae)	hawthorn	berry, flower	regulate blood pressure
Frangula purshiana (DC.) Cooper (Rhamnaceae)	cascara	Bark	Dog B cancer
Galium aparine L. (Rubiaceae)	cleavers	aerial	detoxification
Ganoderma lucidum (Leyss.) (Ganodermataceae)	reishi	Fruiting body	Dog A cancer
Glycyrrhiza glabra L. (Fabaceae)	licorice	Root	Dog B cancer
Iris versicolor L. (Iridaceae)	blue flag	root	Dog A lymphatic drainage
Lavandula officinalis L. (Labiatae)	lavender	flowers	detoxification
Lentinula edodes (Berk.) Pegler (Marasmiaceae)	shiitake	Fruiting body	Dog A cancer
Phytolacca decandra L. (Phytolaccaceae)	poke root	Roots, berries	Dog A cancer
Plantago ovata Forssk. (Plantaginaceae)	psyllium	seeds	Dog B cancer
Rheum palmatum L. (Polygonaceae)	turkey rhubarb	Root, stem	Dogs A & B cancer
Rumex acetosella L. (Polygonaceae)	sheep sorrel	leaf	Dog A cancer
Rumex crispus L. (Polygonaceae)	yellow dock	root	Dog B cancer, detoxification
Salix alba L.(Salicaceae)	white willow	bark	detoxification
Stellaria media (L.) Cyrill. (Caryophyllaceae)	chickweed	aerial parts	detoxification

Stillingia sylvatica Garden ex L., (Euphorbiaceae)	stillingia	root	Dog A lymphatic drainage
Taraxacum officinale (L.) Weber (Asteraceae)	dandelion	root	Dog A lymphatic drainage, detoxification, cancer
Trifolium pratense L. (Fabaceae)	red clover	Aerial parts, flowers	detoxification, cancer, tumour growth in prostate cases
Ulmus fulva Michx. (Ulmaceae) purchased product	slippery elm	bark	Dogs A& B cancer
Urtica dioica L. (Urticaceae)	nettle	leaves	detoxification
Verbascum thapsus L. (Scrophulariaceae)	mullein	Aerial parts	Dog A lymphatic drainage
YUCCA SCHIDIGERA Roezl ex Ortgies (Agavaceae)	yucca	root	detoxification
Zingiber officinale Roscoe (Zingiberaceae)	ginger	Root	Dog B cancer

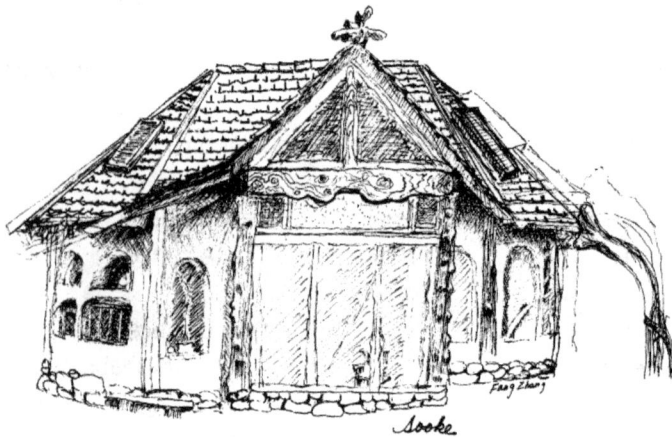

TABLE 15. NON-EXPERIMENTAL VALIDATION OF PLANTS USED FOR CANCER IN PETS IN BRITISH COLUMBIA

Medicinal plant	Validation information	Reference	Validation
Achillea millefolium	*A. millefolium* demonstrated dominant cytotoxicity, with an IC50 value of1422.0 µg/mL against the following human hepatoma cell lines: HepG2/C3A (hepatoblastoma cell line) 430.4 µg/mL against the HA22T/VGH cell line, and (40.7%) inhibitory effect against the SK-HEP-1 cell line. *A. millefolium* had an inhibition percentage of 21.8% against the Hep3B cell line.	Lin et al., 2002	3
Althaea officinalis	*Althaea officinalis* root is traditionally used for its healing mucilage and it is generally recognised as safe (GRAS).	Elmastas et al., 2004; Blumenthal et al., 2000	3
Apium graveolens	*Apium graveolens* has anti-inflammatory activity. Celery seed oil contains p-Mentha-2,8-dien-1-ol, 3-n-butyl phthalide and sedanolide. Activities include (1) induce GST (2) inhibition of BP-induced stomach cancer.	Al-Hindawi et al., 1989; Park and Pezzuto, 2002	3
Arctium lappa	Arctigenin is the active principle of *Arctium lappa* and has significant inhibitory activity against PANC-1 tumor cell growth both *in vitro* and *in vivo*.	Awale et al., 2006	3
Artemisia annua	Oral artemisinin significantly delayed (P<.002) and in some animals prevented (57% of artemisinin-fed versus 96% of the controls developed tumors, P<.01) breast cancer development in rats. In addition, breast tumors in artemisinin-fed rats were significantly fewer (P<.002) and smaller in size (P<.05) compared with controls. This study indicated that artemisinin may be a safe and potent cancer-chemoprevention agent.	Singh and Lai, 2001; Lai and Singh, 2006	4

Berberis vulgaris	Berbamine has been demonstrated to posess significant leukogenic effect, to be anti-hypertensive, anti-arrhythmic and immunosuppressive. Berbamine can inhibit the lymphoproliferative response to ConA and LPS, decrease the PFC numbers to T-dependent antigen (sheep red blood cells; SRBC). Berbamine can decrease the ratio of CD4-positive cells to CD8-positive cells.	Luo et al., 1998	4
Borago officinalis	An *in vitro* study deomstrated that gamolenic acid (oil from the seeds of evening primrose and borage) potentiates the cytotoxicity of paclitaxel and vinorelbime in human breast cancer cell lines.	Shia et al., 2004	4
Crataegus oxyacantha	Hawthorn has antioxidant and cardiotonic activity. The polyphenol fraction of the dried fruits of *Crataegus pinnatifida* showed potential as a cancer chemopreventive agent. The active compounds are uvaol, Ursolic acid and 3-oxo-ursolic acid.	Jayalakshmi and Niranjalim 2004; Habs, 2004; Kao et al., 2007; Min et al., 2000	4
Galium aparine	Asperuloside, an iridoid, has mild laxative and anti-inflammatory activity. The Iranian plant *Galium mite* methanolic extract has antineoplastic activity with an IC50 of 39.8 microg/ml against a K562 leukemia cell line. *Galium mite* caused > 40% apoptosis in K562 and Jurkat cells producing ladder formation. *Galium verum* subsp. v*erum* has antioxidant activity.	Wynn and Marsden, 2003; Amirghofran et al., 2006; Mavi et al., 2004	4
Ganoderma lucidum	*Ganoderma lucidum* is a Chinese herbal medicine used by cancer patients. *In vitro* studies suggested that *Ganoderma lucidum* might impair hemostasis. In a prospective, randomized double-blind study healthy volunteers received *Ganoderma lucidum* capsules 1.5 g (n = 20) or placebo (n = 20) orally daily for 4 wk. *Ganoderma lucidum* ingestion over 4 wk was not associated with impairment of hemostasis. Exogenous	Kwok et al., 2005; Shidoji, Y., Ogawa, H., 2004	3

geranylgeranoic acid (GGA) is a micromolar inducer of apoptosis in human hepatoma-derived cells. *Ganoderma lucidum* whole plant from China has 0.4 µg/g dry wt geranylgeranoic acid (GGA), and a ratio of GGA/ phytanic acid of 0.6.

Glycyrrhiza glabra	Glycyrrhizin, a sweet-tasting triterpenoid saponin, is a major component of licorice root (*Glycyrrhiza glabra* L.). Glycyrrhizin and its aglycone, glycyrrhetinic acid, induce interferon activity and augment natural killer cell activity. Chalcones in licorice possess antiviral activity. Glycyrrhizin also has antiinflammatory properties.	Wynn and Marsden, 2003; Wagner and Jurcic, 2002	3
Iris versicolor	Iris contains flavonoids, benzoquinones and triterpenes. Some flavonoids may enhance the anxiolytic and sedative properties of diazepam and perhaps of natural agonists of the benzodiazepine receptor.	Adams and Garcia, 2006	3
Lavandula officinalis	Perillyl alcohol comes from the essential oils of lavender, peppermint, cherries, sage, and lemongrass. It has shown potential in the treatment of pancreatic cancer.	Lebedeva et al., 2008; Matos et al., 2008	3
Lentinula edodes	Anti-tumour activity is attributed to polysaccharides that activate the immune system and are found in shiitake (*Lentinula edodes*) and reishi (*Ganoderma lucidum*). Their use extended the survival of cancer patients and/or improved the quality of life in patients with advanced cancer. Lentinan, a high molecular weight anti-tumor polysaccharide is found in *Lentinula edodes*. LEM, a protein-bound polysaccharide from *Lentinula edodes* mycelia, exhibits similar immune regulatory effects as Lentinan. Other bioactive components include eritadenine.	Gu and Belury, 2005	3
Phytolacca	Pokeweed antiviral protein, a ribosome-inactivating protein from *Phytolacca*	D'Cruz et al., 2004; Yang et al.,	3

decandra	*americana*, has antiviral activity. It has potent cytotoxic activity once it enters the cytoplasm of a cell but it is incapable of entering cells by itself.	2003	
Plantago ovata	Fiber from *Plantago ovata* had a positive effect on rat colons and it may be beneficial in human inflammatory bowel disease.	Rodrígues-Cabezas et al., 2002	3
Rheum palmatum	Exogenous geranylgeranoic acid (GGA) is a micromolar inducer of apoptosis in human hepatoma-derived cells. GGA and its 4,5-didehydro derivative both inhibit experimental hepato-carcinogenesis and induce differentiation and apoptosis in human hepatoma-derived cell lines. A one-year intake of 4,5-didehydro GGA is effective for prevention of second primary hepatoma and increased the 5-year survival rate in a phase II double-blinded, placebo-controlled clinical trial with relatively low toxicity. GGA is a natural component of dry herbs. *Rheum palmatum* root from China has 1.7 µg/g dry wt geranylgeranoic acid (GGA) and a ratio of GGA/ phytanic acid of 2.8.	Shidoji, Y., Ogawa, H., 2004	3
Rhamnus purshiana/ Frangula purshiana	*R. purshiana* exhibited strong cytotoxicity (IC50 = 381.2 µg/mL), against a PLC/PRF/5 human hepatoma cell line.	Lin et al., 2002	3
R.acetosella, Rumex crispus	*Rumex* is one plant used in Harry M. Hoxsey's (1901-1974) famous cancer elixir. *Rumex crispus* aqueous and methanol extracts show inhibition of HIV reverse transcriptase. *Rumex acetosa* leaf contains the antioxidants catechin and epicatechin.	Vermani and Garg, 2002; Tai and Cheung 2005; Stoggl et al., 2004	2
Salix alba	An extract from the young leaves of *Salix safsaf* delayed the cancer-related deaths of mice by a month. Willow bark extracts have shown anticancer activity when tested on	El-Shemy et al., 2007; Hostanska et al., 2007	3

human colon and lung cancer cell lines.

Stellaria media	A *S. media* crude drug demonstrated strong cytotoxicity, with an IC50 value of 197.6 µg/mL on a Hep3B human hepatoma cell line.	Lin et al., 2002	3
Stillingia sylvatica	The most unstudied ingredient in Harry M. Hoxsey's famous cancer remedy. Roots contain diterpene-esters with possible antitumour activity.	Zick et al., 2006; Adolf and Hecker, 1980; Fine et al., 1988	3
Taraxacum officinale	Exogenous geranylgeranoic acid (GGA) is a micromolar inducer of apoptosis in human hepatoma-derived cells. *Taraxacum officinale* root from Hungary has 0.3 µg/g dry wt geranylgeranoic acid (GGA) and a ratio of GGA/ phytanic acid of 0.8.	Shidoji and Ogawa, 2004	3
Trifolium pratense	Studies on phytoestrogens, such as standardized plant extracts with *in vitro* and *in vivo* estrogenic activity from red clover (*Trifolium pratense* L.), suggest clinical efficacy. It showed photoprotective effects after topical application in hairless mice, reducing photocarcinogenesis. Red clover extracts can stimulate differentiation of human osteoblastic osteosarcoma cells.	Chadwick et al., 2006; Jellinek and Maloney, 2005	3
Ulmus fulva	*Ulmus rubra* has antitumor activity demonstrated through inhibition of proliferation and induction of apoptosis of human breast cancer cells through several mechanisms. An *Ulmus* extract demonstrated *in vitro* antiproliferative activity on cervical, melanoma, breast cancer, and histiocytic lymphoma cell lines.	Jellinek and Maloney, 2005	4
Urtica dioica	The water extract of *Urtica dioica* has significant antioxidant activity against various oxidative systems *in vitro*. It's antioxidant mechanisms can be attributed	Gülçin et al., 2004; Aksu et al., 2008; Celik and Tuluce, 2007;	4

	to phenolic compounds. Nettles consumption was shown to reduce radiation toxicity in cancer treatment. Nettles showed protective effects against carcinogenic chemical induced injury in rats. Nettles aqueous extract showed beneficial effects when incubated with prostate tissue from patients with prostate cancer.	Durak et al., 2004	
Verbascum thapsus	*Verbascum thapsus* crude drug had 31% inhibition (at 2000 μg/mL (IC50)) on a Hep G2/C3a cell line; 69.9 on the HA22T/VGH cell line and 11.6 on the PLC/PRF/5 cell line.	Lin et al., 2002	3
Yucca schidigera	*Yucca schidigera* has a very high level of saponins and phenolic compounds with antioxidant action. One study investigated the antiplatelet mechanisms of four phenolic compounds that had been isolated from the bark of *Y. schidigera* - phenolic compounds (1 to 25 microg/mL) and their extracts decreased platelet adhesion and secretion.	Olas et al., 2005	3
Zingiber officinale	The antioxidant curcumin (a diferuloylmethane), is an	Craig, 1999; Park and Pezzuto, 2002; Kang et al., 2006;	3

effective antiinflammatory agent in humans. The rhizome

of ginger contains curcumin in addition to a dozen phenolic

compounds with antioxidant activity. An ethanol extract of ginger mediated anti-tumor promoting effects in a mouse skin tumorigenesis model. Pre-application of ginger extract on the skin of SENCAR mice resulted in significant inhibition of TPA-induced epidermal ODC, COX and lipoxygenase activity. In a long-term study, ginger extract also significantly protected against skin tumor incidence. 6-gingerol, has wide-ranging pharmacological activities, including inhibition of COX and lipoxygenase activities. Ginger rhizome showed cytotoxicity against ER-negative breast

cancer (MDA-MB-231) of 60 ± 3.3 IC50
(µg/mL) cervix epitheloid (HeLa) 82 ±
3.4IC50 (µg/mL) cell lines.

TABLE 16. MEDICINAL PLANTS OR CLOSELY RELATED PLANTS TO THOSE IN THE BC ETHNOVETERINARY RESEARCH CONTAINING LUTEOLIN (ANTI-CANCER COMPOUND) (DUKE, 1990)

Medicinal plant	Common name	Plant part
Achillea millefolium	yarrow	plant
Apium graveolens	celery	seed, leaf
Artemisia annua , A. drancunculus	sweet wormwood, tarragon	plant
Crataegus laevigata	hawthorn	fruit, bud, leaf
Crataegus monogyna	hawthorn	tissue culture, fruit
Crataegus rhipidophylla	hawthorn	leaf, bud, fruit
Lavandula angustifolia	lavender	plant
Plantago major	plantain	leaf
Plantago ovata	psyllium	leaf
Stellaria media	chickweed	shoot
Taraxacum officinale	dandelion	flower

ETHNOVETERINARY REMEDIES USED IN BRITISH COLUMBIA CANADA FOR ANXIETY, RESPIRATORY AND CARDIAC PROBLEMS IN DOGS AND CATS

Abstract

In 2003 we conducted semi-structured interviews with 60 participants involved in animal health care obtained using a purposive sample. We found that medicinal plants are used to treat a range of conditions in animals. This chapter presents the medicinal plants used to treat anxiety, respiratory and cardiac problems in British Columbia. The following plants were used for asthma: borage (*Borago officinalis* L., Boraginaceae), pumpkin (*Cucurbita pepo* L., Cucurbitaceae), flaxseed oil (*Linum usitatissimum* L., Linaceae), lobelia (*Lobelia inflata* L., Lobeliaceae), mullein (*Verbascum thapsus* L., Scrophulariaceae), and ginger (*Zingiber officinale* Roscoe, Zingiberaceae). Heart problems were treated with balm of Gilead (*Cedronella canariensis* (L.) Willd. ex Webb & Berth, Labiatae), hawthorn (*Crataegus oxyacantha* L., Rosaceae), lady slipper (*Cypripedium calceolus* L., Orchidaceae), horsetail (*Equisetum palustre* L., Equisetaceae), hops (*Humulus lupulus* L., Cannabinaceae), lobelia (*Lobelia inflata* L., Campanulaceae), pine (*Pinus ponderosa* Douglas ex Lawson, Pinaceae), wood betony (Stachys officinalis (L.) Trev., Lamiaceae), valerian (*Valeriana officinalis* L., Valerianaceae), and mistletoe (*Viscum album* L., Loranthaceae). Twenty species of plants were used for motion sickness, anxiety and epilepsy in pets including *Valeriana officinalis*, skullcap (*Scutellaria lateriflora* l., Lamiaceae) and passion flower (*Passiflora incarnata* L. (Passifloraceae). Oatstraw (*Avena sativa* L., Poaceae), wild lettuce *Lactuca muralis* (L.) Fresen., Asteraceae), summer savoury (*Satureja hortensis* L., Lamiaceae) and lady slipper *Cypripedium calceolus* L., Orchidaceae) were the only plants with no known clinical studies to support the ethnoveterinary uses.

Keywords: anxiety; pets; ethnoveterinary medicine; British Columbia

Background

In 2003 research on the ethnoveterinary remedies used in British Columbia, Canada was begun. The medicinal plants used by pet owners, holistic veterinarians and farmers were documented and validated (in a non-experimental way) the medicinal plants.

This chapter presents some if the medicinal plants used to treat anxiety, cardiac and respiratory problems in dogs and cats in British Columbia. This research also records the remedies used to treat anxiety in pets.

2. Materials and methods

The methods are outlined in detail in the introductory chapter.

3. Results

Table 17 summarises the ethnoveterinary remedies used in British Columbia for pets with asthma. Table 18 contains the treatments used in British Columbia for pets with blood pressure and/or cardiac problems. Table 19 lists the plants used for treating anxiety, epilepsy and motion sickness.

Treatment for asthma

A tea is made by steeping 60 ml (¼ cup) dried mullein leaves (*Verbascum thapsus*) in 240 ml boiling water. This is cooled and strained and the resulting liquid given once or twice daily. Two tbsp of tea is recommended for a 10 lb cat. Dogs with asthma are given a purchased lobelia tincture (*Lobelia inflata*) (40 drops of tincture in 240 ml of apple cider vinegar per 23 – 27 kg (50 to 60 lbs bodyweight). Ginger is added (60 ml or ¼ tsp powdered). Ten to 20 drops of this supplemented tincture is used for an asthma attack.

Treatment for cardiac problems in dogs and cats

For cardiac problems a tincture is made of 1 flower bud of hawthorn (*Crataegus oxyacantha*) in 20 cc vodka; this is allowed to stand for at least two weeks. One drop/lb patient bodyweight of this tincture is added daily to the drinking water.

A commercial product is also used. It contains hawthorn berries (*Crataegus oxyacantha*), horsetail (*Equisetum arvense*), valerian (*Valeriana officinalis*), pine needles (*Pinus* sp.), Balm of Gilead, hops (*Humulus lupulus*), lady slipper (*Cypripedium calceolus*), lobelia (*Lobelia inflata*), wood betony (*Stachys officinalis*) and mistletoe (*Viscum album*). The dose used is 1 drop per 10 kg.

Plants used to regulate blood pressure in dogs and cats

A tincture of hawthorn berries and flowers (*Crataegus oxyaantha*) is used for low or high blood pressure. A tincture is made with 60 ml (¼ cup) dried crushed berries and 60 ml (¼ cup) crushed hawthorn flowers added to 2 cups of (500 ml) gin, brandy or rum (1 to 3 drops of the tincture twice a day for 2 weeks). A hawthorn decoction can be used instead 120 ml (½ cup) berries and flowers to 480 ml (2 cups) of water and decocted for 15 minutes). The hawthorn dose is 1 tsp (5 ml) in a little water per 9 kg (20 lb) patient bodyweight every morning and evening before meals for two weeks.

Treatment for anxiety problems in pets

Dogs that show anxiety in various forms are given 5 ml nutritional yeast (1 tsp) on their food and a multi-vitamin for dogs is also given daily. Alternatively pets are given a B complex vitamin as well as a multi-vitamin for cats/ dogs. A multi-compound tincture is put in the dog's food (under 7 kg (15 lbs) bodyweight). Ingredients are 5 ml (1 tsp) each of flowers of chamomile (*Matricaria recutita*), aerial parts of skullcap (*Scutellaria lateriflora*), and leaves of passion flower (*Passiflora incarnata*). One ml (1 tsp) two or three times a day is given in food or water for a couple of months.

A purchased product called Bach Flower Rescue Remedy is used by several respondents for anxiety in pets. Dogs are given 1 - 4 drops, diluted in 50 ml drinking water or drops are given directly in the animal's mouth. Rescue Remedy is also given one hour before or after meals. Cats are given 1 to 4 drops applied to the paw or the back of the neck or the remedy is diluted in 50 ml water before being applied. Anxious show animals are given 1 drop Rescue Remedy on the tongue 20 minutes before going into the show ring. Anxious pets are also given 1 to 2 drops per 18 – 23 kg (40 to 50 lb) patient bodyweight of any of the following purchased tinctures on the tongue: valerian (*Valeriana officinalis*), skullcap (*Scutellaria lateriflora*), hops (*Humulus lupulus*) and passion flower (*Passiflora incarnata*).

Valerian root tincture (*Valeriana officinalis*) (1:5 alcohol) is given to dogs, 1 drop for every 2 kg (5 lb) body weight. The alcohol is evaporated off first. Cats are given 1 or 2 drops of a non-alcoholic tincture. Cats are generally not given alcohol-based tinctures.

Jack Russells were given 20 drops every four hours for several weeks to treat their separation anxiety. A tea can be made with 60 ml (¼ cup) of crushed *Valeriana officinalis* root in 475 ml (2 cups) of water. Dogs are given 30 ml (2 tbsp) of the tea per 9 kg (20 lb) bodyweight every four hours.

Dogs are given the cut dried leaves of dandelions (*Taraxacum officinalis*), 2 – 5 ml (1/2 – 1 tsp) per 4.5 kg (10 lb) bodyweight; this is alternated with alfalfa (*Medicago sativa*), 2 – 5 ml (1/2 – 1 tsp) for every 4.5 kg patient bodyweight, to add minerals and natural plant enzymes to the diet. These plants are only mixed with wet food, or preferably with homemade food. Pets are given Acadian Sea kelp powder, 1 ml (1/8 tsp) per 4.5 kg patient bodyweight. This is added to the diet 2 –3 times a week as a tonic, blood cleanser, for trace minerals and iodine.

Dogs are given rose hip tea, 60 ml rose hips to 475 ml water (¼ cup rose hips to 2 cups of water). Five ml strained tea is given for every 4.5 kg patient bodyweight daily. This tea is a source of vitamin C and bioflavonoids. Dogs are also given garlic (*Allium sativum*), ¼ clove per 23 kg (50 lbs) patient bodyweight added to their raw food diet occasionally.

A 3.6 kg (8 lb) cat that grieved the death of a companion pet was treated with the tinctures below: 10 drops of each purchased tincture listed below, or all of the tinctures are blended and 10 drops of the combined mixture was given. The tinctures were composed of aerial parts of heart's ease (*Viola tricolor*), flowers and berries of hawthorn (*Crataegus oxyacantha*), flowers of chamomile (*Matricaria chamomilla*) or aerial parts of skullcap (*Scutellaria lateriflora*).

Anxious pets are given a diet boost consisting of a tea of dried nettles. The tea is made with 60 ml (¼ cup) nettles to 1 L (2 cups) of water per 23 kg (50 to 55 lbs) bodyweight. The strained tea is put on the food. Alternatively an infusion can be made. Or the nettles can be steamed and 5 ml (1 heaping tsp) given to the dog, twice a week for an indefinite period.

Anxious pets are also given the following alternately added to the food: ginger (*Zingiber officinalis*), oregano (*Origanum* sp.), 1/3 clove garlic (*Allium sativum*), rosemary (*Rosmarinus officinalis*) or summer savoury (*Satureja hortensis*).

One family's cats are given parsley tea (*Petroselinum crispum*) for anxiety. This is made by steeping three bunches (5 to 7 stems) aerial parts in 120 ml (½ cup) of hot water. This is cooled, strained and then an ice cube tray is filled with the resulting liquid. One ice block is put in water for two cats. These cats have become accustomed to this treatment and cry if they don't get it.

Treatment for epilepsy

For epilepsy pets are given a tincture of skullcap (*Scutellaria lateriflora*). Three droppers full of alcoholic tincture (60 drops) are given to a 34 kg (75 lb) dog when the dog showed signs of an impending seizure. The drops are given in divided doses throughout the day (the alcohol was evaporated off before use). The owner said that this lessened the severity and incidence of the seizures. This treatment is also used as a preventative: 20 drops in the food. This treatment is given indefinitely. Another 34 kg (75lb) dog is given half the tincture dose. Dogs are also treated with 1 – 5 ml (¼ to 1 tsp) thiamine orally (medium sized dog) when needed. Also used is 1 ml (¼ tsp) Epsom salts (Magnesium sulphate or oxide) orally at every seizure. Dogs are also given 1 drop essential oil of oregano (*Origanum* sp.) behind the ear to calm them. An olive oil infusion made with St. John's Wort (*Hypericum perforatum*) flowers is applied to anxious pets with a cotton ball.

Treatment for motion sickness

Pets are given a combination formula consisting of 1.4 litres (6 cups) of low-sodium chicken broth or water, 60 ml (¼ cup) skullcap leaves (*Scutellaria lateriflora*), 80 ml (1/3 cup) flowers of chamomile (*Matricaria recutita*), 60 ml (¼ cup) cut leaves and stems of oatstraw (*Avena sativa*), 60 ml (¼ cup) lobelia leaves, 60 ml (¼ cup) packed flowers of hops (*Humulus lupulus*) and 80 ml (1/3 cup) passion flower (*Passiflora incarnata*). The dose used is 15ml (1 tbsp) per 17 kg (25 lb) of body weight of the strained liquid for anxiety, as a sedative or for motion sickness. The strained tea is given at least 1 hour before travel. The tea was frozen for later use in an ice cube tray. The tea ice cubes are stored for up to one year in a freezer bag to prevent freezer burn. A 22.6 kg (50 lb) dog is given a 500 mg ginger capsule half-hour before travelling.

Another pet is treated with a wild lettuce leaf tincture (*Lactuca virosa*) made with 240 ml (1 cup) of wild lettuce. For acute stress 20 drops are given every three hours for a 20 kg (40 - 50 lb) dog. Half the dose is used for a smaller dog. The tincture is put in the inner lip. For a reduced amount of stress the same dose is used twice a day.

4. Discussion

The results of the non-experimental validation of these plant remedies is presented in Table 20.

Crataegus oxyacantha, one of the plants used for heart problems in pets in our study, is included in an Indian commercial product called A.V. Circulo. The herbal combination was was evaluated in isoproterenol induced myocardial damage in rats. A.V. Circulo prevented an increase in serum lysosomal enzyme activity of creatinine phosphokinase, lactate dehydrogenase, and serum glutamate oxaloacetic transaminase in the blood due to isoproterenol administration (Chauhan and Naik, 2005). Craig (1999) reviewed the relevant properties of hawthorn. Flavonoids, oligomeric procyanins and catechins are said to be the active compounds. Hawthorn causes dilation of the smooth muscles of the coronary vessels, increasing blood flow and reducing the tendency for angina. Proanthocyanidins inhibit the biosynthesis of thromboxane A_2. Oral and parenteral administration of oligomeric procyanins from hawthorn produce an increase in coronary blood flow in dogs and cats. Double-blind clinical trials have shown cardiotropic as well as vasodilatory activity. In contrast to other inotropic drugs (drugs that cause muscle contractions) such as epinephrine, amrinon, milrinone and digoxin, hawthorn has a reduced arrhythomogenic risk because unlike the other drugs mentioned it can prolong the effective refractory period (Mashour et al., 1998).

Monoterpenes and sesquiterpenes in the essential oil of valerian contribute to its sedative activity. These compounds can inhibit the catabolism of gamma-aminobutyric acid (GABA). Valerian extracts also interacted at other presynaptic components of GABAergic neurons. Amino acids, GABA, and glutamate, in aqueous extracts of the roots are also active compounds, as is valerenic acid (Block et al., 2004). A valerian extract and a hops-valerian extract (*Humulus lupulus* -*Valeriana officinalis*) exhibited partial agonist activity in an adenosine A(1) receptor assay. The lignan olivil, is a partial agonist to adenosine receptors showing A(1) affinity. Valerian may interact with other drugs such as sedatives, hypnotics, tranquilizers, and anesthetics (Block et al., 2004).

5. Conclusion

Avena sativa, *Lactuca muralis* and *Cypripedium calceolus* were the only plants with no known clinical studies to support the ethnoveterinary uses. Wynn and Marsden (2003) acknowledge that *Avena sativa* is a traditional sedative but there is no listing for the other plants in their work. In contrast hawthorn has many supporting studies and is much prescribed in Europe for heart related ailments (Walker et al., 2006).

References

Akoachere, J.F., Ndip, R.N., Chenwi, E.B., Ndip, L.M., Njock, T.E., Anong ,DN.. 2002.Antibacterial effect of *Zingiber officinale* and *Garcinia kola* on respiratory tract pathogens. East Afr Med J. 79(11):588-92.

Akhondzadeh, S., Kashani, L., Mobaseri, M., Hosseini, S.H., Nikzad, S., Khani, M. 2001. Passionflower in the treatment of opiates withdrawal: a double-blind randomized controlled trial. J Clin Pharm Ther. 26(5):369-73.

Anon, 2000. Berberine monograph. Alternative Medicine Review 5: 175-177.

Avallone, R., Zanoli, P., Puia, G., Kleinschnitz, M., Schreier, P., Baraldi, M. 2000. Pharmacological profile of apigenin, a flavonoid isolated from *Matricaria chamomilla*. *Biochem Pharmacol.* 59 (11):1387-94.

Bandoniene, D., Murkovic, M. 2002. The detection of radical scavenging compounds in crude extract of borage (*Borago officinalis* L.) by using an on-line HPLC-DPPH method. J Biochem Biophys Methods. 53(1-3):45-9.

Bergeron, C., Gafner, S., Clausen, E., Carrier, D.J. 2005. Comparison of the chemical composition of extracts from *Scutellaria lateriflora* using accelerated solvent extraction and supercritical fluid extraction versus standard hot water or 70% ethanol extraction. J Agric Food Chem. 53(8):3076-80.

Block, K.I., Gyllenhaal, C.,Mead, M.N. 2004. Safety and efficacy of herbal sedatives in cancer care. Integr Cancer Ther. 3:128.

Blumenthal, M. 2000. Interactions Between Herbs and Conventional Drugs: Introductory Considerations. In: Herbs—everyday reference for health professionals. Ottawa: Canadian Pharmacists Association and Canadian Medical Association. pp. 9-20, 2000.

Campbell, E.L., Chebib, M., Johnston, G.A. 2004. The dietary flavonoids apigenin and (-)-epigallocatechin gallate enhance the positive modulation by diazepam of the activation by GABA of recombinant GABA(A) receptors. Biochem Pharmacol. 68(8):1631-8.

Chadwick, L.R., Pauli, G.F., Farnsworth, N.R. 2006. The pharmacognosy of *Humulus lupulus* L. (hops) with an emphasis on estrogenic properties. Phytomedicine. 2006; 13:119-31.

Chauhan, G.M., Naik, S.R. 2005. Cardioprotective activity of A.V. Circulo in isoproterenol-induced myocardial necrosis. J Herb Pharmacother. 5(4):51-61.

Cinatl, J., Morgenstern, B., Bauer, G., Chandra, P., Rabenau, H., Doerr, H.W. 2003. Glycyrrhizin, an active component of liquorice roots, and replication of SARS-associated coronavirus. Lancet 361(9374):2045-6.

Craig, W.J. 1999. Health-promoting properties of common herbs. Am J Clin Nutr. 70 (suppl), 491S–9S.

Dirsch, V.M., Vollmar, A.M. 2001. Ajoene, a natural product with non-steroidal anti-inflammatory drug (NSAID)-like properties? Biochem Pharmacol. 61(5):587-93.

Do Monte, F.H., dos Santos, J.G. Jr, Russi, M., Lanziotti, V.M., Leal, L.K., Cunha, G.M. 2004. Antinociceptive and anti-inflammatory properties of the hydroalcoholic extract of stems from *Equisetum arvense* L. in mice. Pharmacol Res. 49(3):239-43.

Dorhoi, A., Dobrean, V., Zahan, M., Virag P., 2006. Modulatory effects of several herbal extracts on avian peripheral blood cell immune responses. Phytother. Res. 20, 352–358.

Duke, J. A. 2000. Phytochemical and Ethnobotanical Databases. USDA-ARS-NGRL, Beltsville Agricultural Research Center, Beltsville, Maryland, USA.

Duncan, K.L., Hare, W.R., Buck, W.B. 1997. Malignant hyperthermia-like reaction secondary to ingestion of hops in five dogs. J Am Vet Med Assoc 210: 51-4.

Ferguson, E.A., Littlewood, J.D., Carlotti, D-N., Grover, R., Nuttall T. 2006. Management of canine atopic dermatitis using the plant extract PYM00217: a randomized, double-blind, placebo-controlled clinical study. European Society of Veterinary Dermatology 17: 236–243.

Gürbüz, I., Üstün, O., Yeşilada, E., Sezik, E., Akyürek, N. 2002. *In vivo* gastroprotective effects of five Turkish folk remedies against ethanol-induced lesions. J Ethnopharmacol. 83:241-4.

Gülçin, I., Küfrevioğlu, O.I., Oktay, M., Büyükokuroğlu, M.E. 2004. Antioxidant, antimicrobial, antiulcer and analgesic activities of nettle (*Urtica dioica* L.). J Ethnopharmacol. 90(2-3): 205-15.

Gurley, B.J., Gardner, S.F., Hubbard, M.A., Williams, D.K., Gentry, W.B., Khan, I,A,, Shah, A. 2005. *In vivo* effects of goldenseal, kava kava, black cohosh, and valerian on human cytochrome P450 1A2, 2D6, 2E1, and 3A4/5 phenotypes. Clin Pharmacol Ther. 77:415-26.

Gurman, E.G., Bagirova, E.A., Storchilo, O.V. 1992. The effect of food and drug herbal extracts on the hydrolysis and transport of sugars in the rat small intestine under different experimental conditions. Fiziol Zh SSSR Im I M Sechenova. 78(8):109-16. Article in Russian.

Habeck, M. 2003. Mistletoe compound enters clinical trials. Drug Discov Today 8:52-3.

Hajhashemi, V., Sadraei, H., Ghannadi, A.R., Mohseni, M. 2000. Antispasmodic and anti-diarrhoeal effect of *Satureja hortensis* L. essential oil. J Ethnopharmacol. 71(1-2):187-92.

Hajhashemi, V., Ghannadi, A., Pezeshkian, S.K. 2002. Antinociceptive and anti-inflammatory effects of *Satureja hortensis* L. extracts and essential oil. J Ethnopharmacol. 82(2-3): 83-7.

Harbige, L.S., Fisher, B.A. 2001. Dietary fatty acid modulation of mucosally-induced tolerogenic immune responses. Proc Nutr Soc. 60(4),449-56.

Holetz, F.B., Pessini, G.L., Sanches, N.R., Coretez, D. A.G., Nakamuram C.V., Filho, B.P.D., 2002. Screening of some plants used in the Brazilian folk medicine for the treatment of infectious diseases. Mem Inst Oswaldo Cruz, 97, 1027-1031.

Hu, C., Kitts, D.D. 2004. Luteolin and luteolin-7-O-glucoside from dandelion flower suppress iNOS and COX-2 in RAW264.7 cells. Mol Cell Biochem. 265(1-2):107-13.

Iauk, L., Costanzo, R., Caccamo, F., Rapisarda, A., Musumeci, R., Milazzo, I., Blandino, G. 2006. Activity of *Berberis aetnensis* root extracts on Candida strains. Fitoterapia. 78(2):159-61.

Jaber, R. 2002. Respiratory and allergic diseases: from upper respiratory tract infections to asthma. Prim Care. 29(2):231-61.

Jakovljevic, V., Raskovic, A., Popovic, M., Sabo, J. 2002. The effect of celery and parsley juices on pharmacodynamic activity of drugs involving cytochrome P450 in their metabolism. Eur J Drug Metab Pharmacokinet. 27(3):153-6.

Jimenez-Arellanes, A., Meckes, M., Ramirez, R., Torres, J., Luna-Herrera, J. 2003. Activity against multidrug-resistant *Mycobacterium tuberculosis* in Mexican plants used to treat respiratory diseases. Phytother Res. 17:903-8.

Johnson, V.J., He, Q., Osuchowski, M.F., Sharma, R.P. 2003. Physiological responses of a natural antioxidant flavonoid mixture, silymarin, in BALB/c mice: III. Silymarin inhibits T-lymphocyte function at low doses but stimulates inflammatory processes at high doses. Planta Med. 69(1):44-9.

Kovacs, E., Kuehn, J.J. 2002. Measurements of IL-6, soluble IL-6 receptor and soluble gp130 in sera of B-cell lymphoma patients. Does *Viscum album* treatment affect these parameters? Biomed Pharmacother. 56:152-8.

Lans, C., Harper, T., Georges, K., Bridgewater, E. 2001. Medicinal and ethnoveterinary remedies of hunters in Trinidad. BMC Alternative and Complementary Medicine 1:10.

Lans, C., Turner, N., Brauer, G., Lourenco, G., Georges, K. 2006. Ethnoveterinary medicines used for horses in Trinidad and in British Columbia, Canada. Journal of Ethnobology and Ethnomedicine 2:31.

Lee, H.S., Kim, S.K., Han, J.B., Choi, H.M., Park, J.H., Kim, E.C., Choi, M.S., An, H.J., Um, J.Y., Kim, H.M., Min, B.I. 2006. Inhibitory effects of *Rumex japonicus* Houtt. on the development of atopic dermatitis-like skin lesions in NC/Nga mice. Br J Dermatol. 155:33-8.

Lim, D.Y., Kim, Y.S., Miwa, S. 2004. Influence of lobeline on catecholamine release from the isolated perfused rat adrenal gland. Auton Neurosci. 110:27-35.

Lopez-Garcia, R.E., Hernandez-Perez, M., Rabanal, R.M., Darias, V., Martin-Herrera, D., Arias, A., Sanz, J. 1992. Essential oils and antimicrobial activity of two varieties of *Cedronella canariensis* (L.) W. et B. J Ethnopharmacol. 36:207-11.

Luo, C.N., Lin, X., Li, W.K., Pu, F., Wang, L.W., Xie, S.S., Xiao, P.G. 1998. Effect of berbamine on T-cell mediated immunity and the prevention of rejection on skin transplants in mice. J Ethnopharmacol. 59:211-5.

Mashour, N.H., George, I.L., Frishman, W.H. 1998. Herbal medicine for the treatment of cardiovascular disease. Arch Intern Med. 158: 2225 – 2234.

Mekhfi, H., Haouari, M.E., Legssyer, A., Bnouham, M., Aziz, M., Atmani, F., Remmal, A., Ziyyat, A. 2004. Platelet anti-aggregant property of some Moroccan medicinal plants. Journal of Ethnopharmacology 94(2-3): 317-22.

Moss, M., Cook, J., Wesnes, K., Duckett, P. 2003. Aromas of rosemary and lavender essential oils differentially affect cognition and mood in healthy adults. Int J Neurosci. 113(1):15-38.

Nagle, T.M., Torres, S.M., Horne, K.L., Grover, R., Stevens, M.T. 2001. A randomized, double-blind, placebo-controlled trial to investigate the efficacy and safety of a Chinese herbal product (P07P) for the treatment of canine atopic dermatitis.Vet Dermatol 12(5):265-74.

Oh, H., Kim, D.H., Cho, J.H., Kim, Y.C. 2004. Hepatoprotective and free radical scavenging activities of phenolic petrosins and flavonoids isolated from *Equisetum arvense*. J Ethnopharmacol. 95(2-3):421-4.

Peredery, O., Persinger, M.A. 2004. Herbal treatment following post-seizure induction in rat by lithium pilocarpine: *Scutellaria lateriflora* (Skullcap), *Gelsemium sempervirens* (Gelsemium) and *Datura stramonium* (Jimson Weed) may prevent development of spontaneous seizures. Phytother Res. 18(9):700-5.

Peeters, E., Driessen, B., Steegmans, R., Henot, D., Geers, R. 2004. Effect of supplemental tryptophan, vitamin E, and a herbal product on responses by pigs to vibration. J Anim Sci. 82:2410-20.

Philipov, S., Istatkova, R., Ivanovska, N., Denkova, P., Tosheva, K., Navas, H., Villegas, J. 1998. Phytochemical study and antiinflammatory properties of *Lobelia laxiflora* L. Z Naturforsch [C]. 53(5-6):311-7.

Rabbani, M., Sajjadi, S.E., Zarei, H.R. 2003. Anxiolytic effects of *Stachys lavandulifolia* Vahl on the elevated plus-maze model of anxiety in mice. *Journal of Ethnopharmacology* 89 (2-3): 271-6.

Reisman, J., Schachter, H.M., Dales, R.E., Tran, K., Kourad, K., Barnes, D., Sampson, M., Morrison A, Gaboury I, Blackman J. 2006. Treating asthma with omega-3 fatty acids: where is the evidence? A systematic review BMC Complement Altern Med. 19; 6:26.

Rimkiene, S., Ragazinskiene, O., Savickiene, N. 2003. The cumulation of wild pansy (*Viola tricolor* L.) accessions: the possibility of species preservation and usage in medicine. Medicina (Kaunas). 39(4):411-6.

Schaefermeyer, G., Schaefermeyer, H. 1998. Treatment of pancreatic cancer with *Viscum album* (Iscador): a retrospective study of 292 patients 1986 – 1996. Complementary Therapies in Medicine 6:172 – 177.

Schütz, K., Carle, R., Schieber, A. 2006. Taraxacum--a review on its phytochemical and pharmacological profile. J Ethnopharmacol. 107(3):313-23.

Smith, H. 1928. Materia medica of the Bella Coola and neighbouring tribes of British Columbia. National Museum of Canada Bulletin, No. 56, King's Printers, Ottawa, Ont., pp 47 – 68.

Smith, H.H. 1933. Ethnobotany of the Forest Potawatomi Indians. Bulletin of the Public Museum of the City of Milwaukee. 7(1): 1 – 230. Milwaukee, Wis.

Spelman, K., Burns, J., Nichols, D., Winters, N., Ottersberg, S., Tenborg, M. 2006. Modulation of cytokine expression by traditional medicines: a review of herbal immunomodulators. Altern Med Rev. 11(2):128-50.

Spinella, M. 2002. The importance of pharmacological synergy in psychoactive herbal medicines. Altern Med Rev. 7(2):130-7.

Stamatis, G., Kyriazopoulos, P., Golegou, S., Basayiannis, A., Skaltsas, S., Skaltsa, H. 2003. *In vitro* anti-*Helicobacter pylori* activity of Greek herbal medicines. *Journal of Ethnopharmacology* 88 (2-3): 175-9.

Stochmal, A., Piacente, S., Pizza, C., De Riccardis, F., Leitz, R., Oleszek, W. 2001. Alfalfa (*Medicago sativa* L.) flavonoids. 1. Apigenin and luteolin glycosides from aerial parts. J Agric Food Chem. 49(2):753-8.

Subarnas, A., Oshima, Y., Sidik, O.Y. 1992. An antidepressant principle of *Lobelia inflata* L. (Campanulaceae). J Pharm Sci. 81(7):620-1.

Tabuti, J., Dhillion, S., Kaare, L. 2003. Ethnoveterinary medicines for cattle (*Bos indicus*) in Bulamogi county, Uganda: Plant species and mode of use. J Ethnopharmacol 88: 279 – 286.

Tanaka, Y., Kikuzaki, H., Fukuda, S., Nakatani, N. 2001. Antibacterial compounds of licorice against upper airway respiratory tract pathogens. J Nutr Sci Vitaminol 47 (3): 270-3.

Turker, U., Camper, N.D. 2002. Biological activity of common mullein, a medicinal plant. Journal of Ethnopharmacology 82:117 – 125.

Tunón, H., Olavsdotter, C., Bohlin, L. 1995. Evaluation of anti-inflammatory activity of some Swedish medicinal plants. Inhibition of prostaglandin biosynthesis and PAF-induced exocytosis. Journal of Ethnopharmacology 48: 61-76.

Uzun, E., Sariyar, G., Adsersen, A., Karakoc, B., Ötük, G., Oktayoglu, E., Pirildar, S. 2004. Traditional medicine in Sakarya province (Turkey) and antimicrobial activities of selected species. J Ethnopharmacol. 95:287-96.

Wang, X., Jia, W., Aihua Zhao, A., Wang, X. 2006. Anti-influenza agents from plants and Traditional Chinese Medicine. Phytother. Res. 20: 335–341.

Walker AF, Marakis G, Simpson E, Hope JL, Robinson PA, Hassanein M, Simpson HC. 2006. Hypotensive effects of hawthorn for patients with diabetes taking prescription drugs: a randomised controlled trial. Br J Gen Pract. 56(527):437-43.

Wolfson, P., Hoffmann, D.L. 2003. An investigation into the efficacy of *Scutellaria lateriflora* in healthy volunteers. Altern Ther Health Med. 9(2):74-8.

Wynn, S.G., Marsden, S.A. 2003. Manual of Natural Veterinary Medicine: Science and Tradition. Mosby: St Louis.

Zanoli, P., Rivasi, M., Zavatti, M., Brusiani, F., Baraldi, M. 2005. New insight in the neuropharmacological activity of *Humulus lupulus* L. J Ethnopharmacol. 102:102-6.

Zheng, W., Wang, S.Y. 2001. Antioxidant activity and phenolic compounds in selected herbs. J Agric Food Chem. 49(11):5165-70.

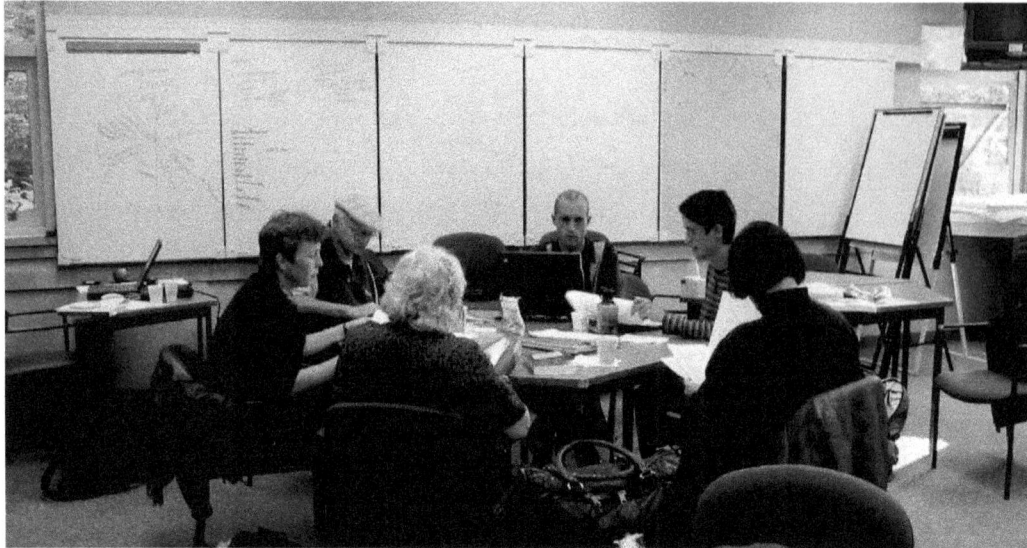

Herbalists, veterinarians, farmers and animal caretakers at the workshop

Goats, Sheep, Poultry	Jan Bevan *	Hornby Island
Dairy goats	Jill Tyndale *	Mount Lehman
Goats	Willi Boepple *	Highlands
Sheep, turkeys	Lorna Kearney *	Duncan
Herbalists	CHGC *	Port Alberni
Horses	Margaret Hall *	Chilliwack
Horses	Alvina Helfenstein *	Delta
Herbalist	Kerry Hackett *	Ontario
Herbalist	Claudia Sheils *	Victoria
DVM	Dr. Tonya Khan *	Vancouver
DVM	Dr. Donna Kelleher *	Seattle

TABLE 17. ETHNOVETERINARY REMEDIES USED IN BRITISH COLUMBIA FOR PETS WITH ASTHMA

Scientific name	Common name	Plant part used
Borago officinalis L. (Boraginaceae)	borage	oil
Cucurbita pepo L. (Cucurbitaceae)	pumpkin	oil
Linum usitatissimum L. (Linaceae)	flax seed	oil
Lobelia inflata L. (Lobeliaceae)	lobelia	aerial parts
Verbascum thapsus L. (Scrophulariaceae)	mullein	dried leaves
Zingiber officinale Roscoe (Zingiberaceae)	ginger	rhizome

TABLE 18. TREATMENTS USED IN BRITISH COLUMBIA FOR PETS WITH CARDIAC AND BLOOD PRESSURE PROBLEMS

Scientific name	Common name	Part used
Cedronella canariensis (L.) Willd. ex Webb & Berth	Balm of Gilead	leaf buds
Crataegus oxyacantha L. (Rosaceae)	hawthorn	flower bud, berries
Cypripedium calceolus L. (Orchidaceae)	lady slipper	root
Equisetum palustre L. (Equisetaceae)	horsetail	stems
Humulus lupulus L. (Cannabinaceae)	hops	stroibles
Lobelia inflata L. (Campanulaceae)	lobelia	aerial part
Pinus ponderosa Douglas ex Lawson (Pinaceae)	pine	Needles
Stachys officinalis (L.) Trev. (Lamiaceae)	wood betony	aerial part
Valeriana officinalis L. (Valerianaceae)	valerian	root
Viscum album L. (Loranthaceae)	mistletoe	leaves, twigs

TABLE 19. ETHNOVETERINARY REMEDIES IN BRITISH COLUMBIA FOR DOGS AND CATS WITH ANXIETY, EPILEPSY OR MOTION SICKNESS

Scientific name	Common name	Plant part used	Use
Allium sativum L. (Alliaceae)	garlic	clove	anxiety, dietary supplement for motion sickness
Avena sativa (Poaceae)	oatstraw	leaves & stems	motion sickness
Crataegus oxyacantha L. (Rosaceae)	hawthorn	flowers & berries	anxiety
Humulus lupulus L. (Cannabinaceae)	hops	flowers	motion sickness
Hypericum perforatum L. (Hypericaceae)	St. John's wort	flowers	anxiety
Lactuca muralis (L.) Fresen. (Asteraceae)	wild lettuce	leaf	acute stress
Lobelia inflata L. (Campanulaceae)	lobelia	leaves	motion sickness
Matricaria chamomilla L. (Compositae)	chamomile	flowers	anxiety, motion sickness
Medicago sativa L. (Fabaceae)	alfalfa	leaves	anxiety
Origanum sp. (Lamiaceae)	oregano	leaves	anxiety, Dietary supplement for motion sickness
Passiflora incarnata L. (Passifloraceae)	passion flower	leaves	anxiety, motion sickness
Petroselinum crispum (Apiaceae)	parsley	aerial parts	anxious cat treatment
Rosmarinus officinalis L. (Lamiaceae)	rosemary	aerial parts	dietary supplement for motion sickness
Satureja hortensis L. (Lamiaceae)	summer savoury	leaves	dietary supplement for motion sickness
Scutellaria lateriflora L. (Lamiaceae)	skullcap	aerial parts	anxiety, motion sickness, epilepsy
Taraxacum officinale (L.) Weber (Asteraceae)	dandelion	leaves	anxiety
Urtica dioica L. (Urticaceae)	nettles	Roots, leaves	dietary supplement for motion sickness
Valeriana officinalis L. (Valerianaceae)	valerian	root	anxiety, motion sickness
Viola tricolour L. (Violaceae)	heart's ease	aerial parts	anxiety
Zingiber officinalis Roscoe (Zingiberaceae)	ginger	rhizome	dietary supplement for motion sickness

TABLE 20. NON-EXPERIMENTAL VALIDATION OF PLANTS USED FOR ANXIETY, CARDIAC AND RESPIRATORY PROBLEMS IN PETS IN BRITISH COLUMBIA

Medicinal plant	Validation information	Reference	Validation score
Allium sativum	Garlic was given to pets for anxiety and as a dietary supplement for motion sickness. Ajoene was shown to dose-dependently inhibit the release of LPS (1 microg/mL)-induced prostaglandin E(2) in RAW 264.7 macrophages (IC(50) value: 2.4 microM). This effect was found to be due to an inhibition of COX-2 enzyme activity by ajoene (IC(50) value: 3.4 microM). Ajoene did not reduce COX-2 expression, but increased LPS-induced COX-2 protein and mRNA expression compared to LPS-stimulated cells only. The non-steroidal anti-inflammatory drug indomethacin was shown to act similarly in LPS-activated RAW 264.7 cells.	Dirsch and Vollmar, 2001	3
Avena sativa	*Avena sativa* is used for motion sickness in pets and this is based on the folk medicinal use but no clinical resarch supports this claim. *Avena sativa* has at least eight compounds with sedative activity.	Duke, 2000	3
Borago officinalis	Borage was used for asthma in our study. The dominant antioxidative compound in the crude extract of borage leaves was identified as rosmarinic acid. Borage oil is rich in n-6 PUFA, of which gamma-linolenic acid is rapidly	Bandoniene and Murkovic, 2002 ; Harbige and Fisher, 2001	3

metabolised to longer-chain n-6 PUFA, which enhanced immune system functions, and may be useful in autoimmune disease.

Cedronella canariensis	Balm of Gilead was used for heart problems in our study.	Lopez-Garcia et al., 2002	3

The qualitative and quantitative determination of the essential oils of the aerial part of two varieties of *Cedronella canariensis* (L.) W. et B., namely, *C. canariensis* var. canariensis and *C. canariensis* var. anisata found antimicrobial activity in both oils. The noteworthy inhibition exhibited against *Bordetella bronchiseptica* and *Cryptococcus albidus* may justify the popular use of these plants in the treatment of certain diseases of the respiratory tract.

Crataegus oxyacantha	Hawthorn was used for heart problems and anxiety in pets in our study.	Blumenthal, 2000; Craig, 2007	4

Flowers of *Crataegus* spp., with leaves (and fruits) may enhance the effects of cardiac glycosides and have been used with such drugs in German clinical medicine to reduce the risk of toxic effects. Hawthorn has also been used with digitalis. Hawthorn procyanidins have been found to increase the coronary artery dilatation effect caused by theophylline, caffeine, papaverine, sodium nitrate, adenosine and epinephrine. Hawthorn has increased barbiturate-induced sleeping times. Proanthocyanidins are the active principles in the flower heads of hawthorn (*Crataegus oxyacantha*). These substances were reported to inhibit the biosynthesis of thromboxane

A2. Patients with chronic heart disease who were given 600 mg/d of a hawthorn extract had lower blood pressure and heart rates and less shortness of breath when exercising compared with subjects not receiving hawthorn.

Cypripedium calceolus	Lady slipper is used to treat pets with heart problems. It is a traditional folk medicine but little scientific work has been done on the orchid.		2
Cucurbita pepo	*Cucurbita pepo* oil is used for asthma in pets. Given the interplay between pro-inflammatory omega-6 fatty acids, and the less pro-inflammatory omega-3 fatty acids, it has been suggested that omega-3 fatty acids found in pumpkin oil could play a key role in treating or preventing asthma.	Reisman et al., 2006; Jaber, 2002	3
Equisetum palustre	Horsetail is an ethnoveterinary remedy for heart problems. There are hepatoprotective and antioxidative principles in the aerial parts of *Equisetum arvense*. The hydroalcoholic extract of stems from *Equisetum arvense* produced an antinociceptive effect when assessed in chemical models of nociception.	Uzun et al., 2004 ; Oh et al., 2004 ; do Monte et al., 2004	3
Humulus lupulus	*Humulus lupulus* is used for heart problems and motion sickness in our study. There was one case of four greyhounds dying after ingesting spent hops. *Humulus lupulus* CO_2 extract and its fraction containing alpha-acids have 2 effects:(a) a pentobarbital sleep-enhancing property without influencing the motor behavior of rats; (b) an antidepressant activity. The same	Duncan et al., 1997 ; Zanoli et al., 2005 ; Chadwick et al., 2004	3

	effects were elicited by the administration of the *Humulus lupulus* fraction containing alpha-acids. A mild sedative in phytomedicine; hops (*Humulus lupulus*) has been investigated for its estrogenic activity (known and more potent estrogen (±)-8-prenylnaringenin and the weaker but more abundant flavanone isoxanthohumol).		
Hypericum perforatum	St John's Wort was used for anxiety in pets.	Spinella, 2002; Blumenthal, 2000	4
	There are synergistic actions in St. John's wort (*Hypericum perforatum*), kava kava (*Piper methysticum*), and valerian (*Valeriana officinalis*). In a clinical study with the valepotriate fraction, reduction of the adverse effects of simultaneously administered alcohol was observed, with a dose-dependent increase in the ability to concentrate.		
Lactuca muralis	*Lactuca muralis* was used for acute stress in pets.	Smith, 1933	2
	Lactuca spicata was used medicinally by the Forest Potawatomi.		
Linum usitatissimum	Asthma in pets is treated with flax.	Jaber, 2002	3
	Patients with asthma and allergic rhinitis may benefit from hydration and a diet low in sodium, omega-6 fatty acids, and trans fatty acids, but high in omega-3 fatty acids (pumpkin, and flax seeds).		

Lobelia inflata	Heart problems and motion sickness in pets are treated with lobelia.	Philipov et al., 1998; Subarnas et al., 1992	3
	Lobelia laxiflora has antiinflammatory activity. A crude methanolic extract of the leaves *of Lobelia inflata* showed antidepressant activity in mice.		
Matricaria chamomilla	*Matricaria chamomilla* is used for anxiety and motion sickness in pets.	Avallone et al., 2000	3
	Apigenin from *Matricaria chamomilla* injected i.p. in rats reduced locomotor activity, but did not demonstrate anxiolytic, myorelaxant, or anticonvulsant activities.		
Medicago sativa	Anxiety in pets is treated with *Medicago sativa*.	Stochmal et al., 2001; Campbell et al., 2004	3
	The flavonoids apigenin and luteolin glycosides are found in the aerial parts. Apigenin (1 microM) enhanced the modulatory action of diazepam (3 microM) on the activation by GABA (5 microM) of recombinant human alpha1beta2gamma2L GABA(A) receptors by up to 22%.		
Origanum sp.	Oregano was used for anxiety and as a dietary supplement for motion sickness.	Zheng and Wang, 2001	3
	Rosmarinic acid was the predominant phenolic compound found in *Origanum* x *majoricum*.		
Passiflora incarnata	Anxiety and motion sickness in pets is treated with passion flower.		**4**
	Passiflora incarnata extract shows efficacy in the management of anxiety and has an anxiolytic effect.		
Petroselinum crispum	Parsley is used to treat anxious cats.	Jakovljevic et al., 2002	3
	In mice pretreated with parsley juices a prolonged action of pentobarbital with respect to control was observed		

(statistically significant). Parsley juice pretreatment increased and prolonged the analgesic action of aminopyrine and paracetamol.

Pinus contorta	Pine needles are used for heart problems.	Smith, 1933; Tunón et al. 1995	3
	The pitch of *Pinus banksiana* and *Pinus trobus* from the wood and bark were used by the Forest Potawatomi as ointments. The leaves were used to clear the lungs of congestion. They use the leaves of *Pinus resinosa* as a reviver. Several derivatives of abietic acid (a diterpenoid) have been isolated from the needles of *Pinus sylvestris.*		
Rosmarinus officinalis	Rosemary is used for motion sickness in pets.	Moss et al., 2003	3
	Rosemary essential oil produced a significant enhancement of performance for overall quality of memory and secondary memory factors in a group of volunteers (144 divided into 3 groups), but also produced an impairment of speed of memory compared to the control (no odour). The control group was significantly less content than the rosemary group following the completion of the cognitive assessment battery.		
Satureja hortensis	Summer savoury is used for motion sickness in pets.	Hajhashemi et al., 2000; 2002	3
	Satureja hortensis has antinociceptive and anti-inflammatory effects and its activity may not involve opioid and adenosine receptors. In addition to antispasmodic activity *in vitro*, the essential oil of this plant at a dose of 0.1 ml/100 g inhibited castor oil induced diarrhoea in mice.		
Scutellaria	Skullcap was used for anxiety, motion	Wolfson and	4

lateriflora	sickness and epilepsy in pets.	Hoffman, 2003; Bergeron et al., 2005; Peredery and Persinger, 2004	
	The aqueous extract of skullcap was used by North American Indians as a nerve tonic and for its sedative and diuretic properties. A double blind, placebo-controlled study of healthy subjects demonstrated noteworthy anxiolytic effects. Flavonoids and amino acids may be responsible for its anxiolytic activity. Epilepsy was induced in male rats and then they were given one of three herbal treatments. There were one other group and a tap water control. Rats that received a weak solution of the three herbal fluid extracts of *Scutellaria lateriflora* (skullcap), *Gelsemium sempervirens* (gelsemium) and *Datura stramonium* (jimson weed) displayed no seizures during treatment while all the other groups had seizures. When the herbal treatment was stopped, the rats had comparable numbers of spontaneous seizures as the controls.		
Stachys officinalis	Pets with heart problems are given wood betony.	Rabbani et al., 2003; Stamatis et al., 2003	3
	The hydroalcoholic extract of Stachys lavandulifolia showed anxiolytic effects with lower sedative activity than diazepam. The essential oil of Stachys lavandulifolia, at doses of up to 100 mg/kg, did not have any significant effects on mice behaviour on the elevated plus-maze model of anxiety. Aqueous 70% methanol extracts of Stachys alopecuros inhibited the growth of Helicobacter pylori -a Gram-negative bacteria that colonizes the gastric lining.		
Taraxacum officinale	Dandelions are used for anxious pets.	Schutz et al., 2006 ; Hu and	3

A review paper lists the various activities of the plant: diuretic, choleretic, anti-inflammatory, anti-oxidative, anti-carcinogenic, analgesic, anti-hyperglycemic, anti-coagulatory and prebiotic effects. Luteolin and luteolin-7-O-glucoside at concentrations less than 20 microM, significantly ($p < 0.05$) suppressed the productions of nitric oxide and prostaglandin E2 (PGE2) in bacterial lipopolysaccharide activated-mouse macrophage RAW264.7 cells without cytotoxicity. The inhibitory effects were attributed to the suppression of both inducible nitric oxide synthase (iNOS) and cyclooxygenase-2 (COX-2) protein expression. Similar suppression for both inducible enzymes was also found with the ethyl acetate fraction of dandelion flower extract which contained 10% luteolin and luteolin-7-O-glucoside.

Urtica dioica	Dietary supplement for motion sickness in dogs.	Gülçin et al., 2004	3
Valeriana officinalis	Nettles have many medicinal properties. Valerian is used for heart problems, anxiety and motion sickness in pets. Sedafit is a commercial herbal product containing *Valeriana officinalis* L. and *Passiflora incarnata* L. as active components. Sedafit demonstrated sedative and antianxiety effects when tested in three experiments on the stress response in pigs during transport simulation. Phytochemical-mediated modulation of cytochrome P450 (CYP) activity may be responsible for many herb-drug interactions. However this study showed that valerian does not produce CYP-mediated herb-drug interactions.	Peeters et al., 2004 ; Gurley et al., 2005	4
Viola tricolor	*Viola tricolor* is used for anxiety in pets.	Rimkiene et al., 2003; Gurman	3

	Viola tricolor L., has traditionally been used for respiratory problems. It is an ingredient in antitussives, cholagogues, dermatological medicines, roborants and tonics, alternatives, and anti-phlebitis remedies. There is a report that the plant reduces glucose transport.	et al., 1992
Viscum album	Mistletoe is used for heart problems in pets.	Kovacs 2002, Schaefermeyer and Schaefermeyer, 1998; Gurbuz et al., 2002	3

A *Viscum album* extract is used as an immunomodulator for malignant disorders and can be used either alone or in addition to chemo- or radiotherapy. None of 15 patients with Non-Hodgkin's lymphoma with short-term treatment of *Viscum album* extract (1-15 months) had alterations of Interleukin-6 (IL-6) values. IL-6 can be involved in lymphoid malignancies. Twelve patients having long term treatment with the extract (2 – 14 years) had a significant decrease in IL-6 values compared to controls. There were more patients in continuous complete remission in the long-term *Viscum album* group than the short term group. A retrospective analysis showed that the survival rate of 292 patients treated at the Lukas Clinic in Switzerland with the same *Viscum album* extract was better or in the upper ranges of survival times reported in the literature. Three of six rat stomachs were protected from EtOH ulcerogenesis by a herbareous part *Viscum album* decoction.

Zingiber officinale

Ginger was used for asthma and motion sickness in pets.   Akoachere   3

et al., 2002

Zingiber officinale had antibacterial activity on four respiratory tract pathogens- *Staphylococcus aureus*,

Streptococcus pyogenes, Streptococcus pneumoniae and *Haemophilus influenzae.*

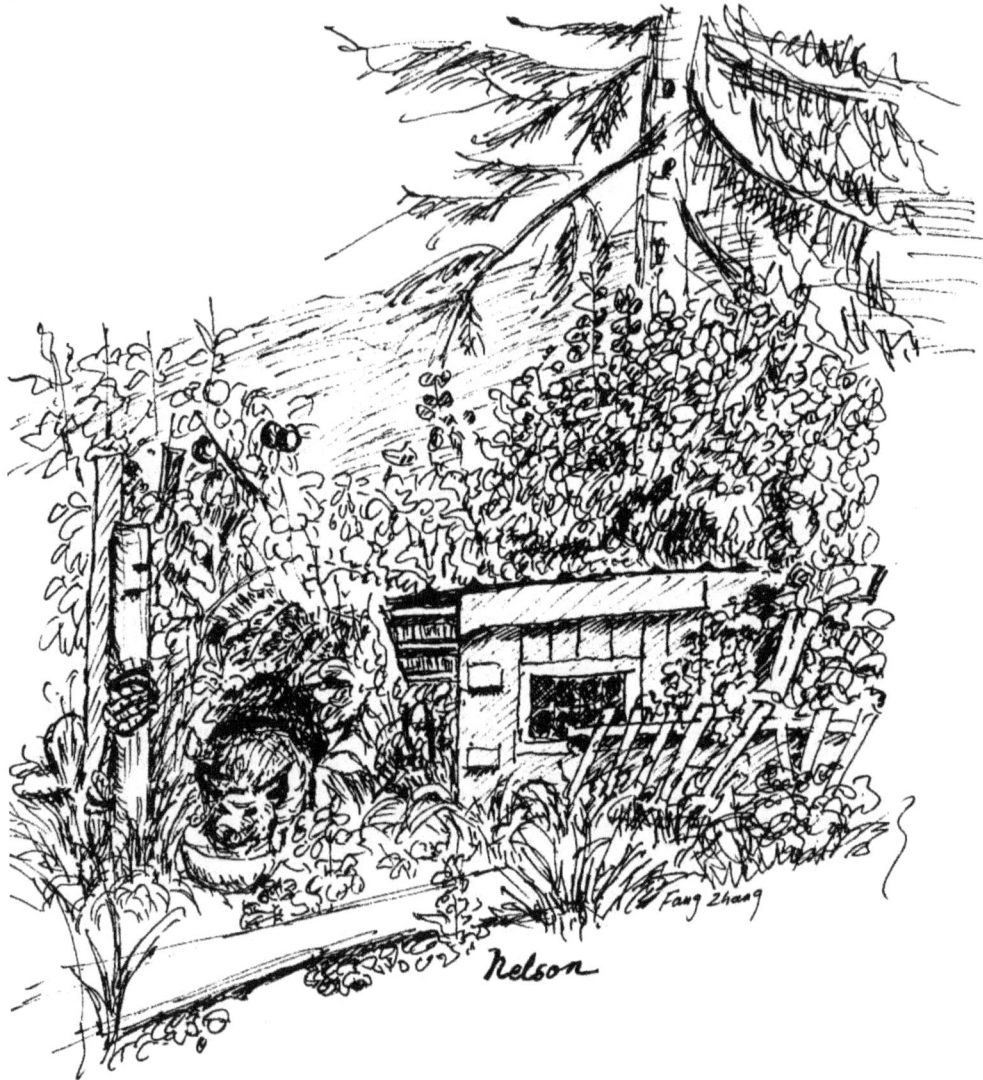

Fang Zhang

Nelson

Abstract

The use of medicinal plants for specific viral and bacterial diseases in pets in British Columbia is addressed in this chapter.

The following plants are used instead of an antibiotic: *Arctostaphylos uva-ursi* (L.) Spreng, *Actaea racemosa* L. var. *racemosa*, *Astragalus membranaceus* (Fisch.), *Hydrastis canadensis* L., *Ulmus fulva* Michx. and *Usnea longissima* Ach. The following plants are used for infectious tracheobronchitis: *Allium sativum* L., *Althaea officinalis* L., *Berberis aquifolium* Pursh./ *Mahonia aquifolium*, *Tussilago farfara* L. and *Verbascum thapsus* L.,*Calendula officinalis* L.,*Plantago major* L., *Stellaria media* (L.) Cyrill., and *Trifolium pratense* . An unidentifed virus was treated with *Crataegus oxycantha* (Rosaceae) and *Echinacea purpurea* (L.) Moench (Asteraceae). *Campylobacter jejuni* (dog show crud) is treated with *Echinacea purpurea* (L.) Moench, *Glycyrrhiza glabra* L., *Mahonia nervosa* (Pursh) Nutt and *Hydrastis canadensis* L. Parvovirus was treated with *Hydrastis canadensis* L, *Astragalus membranaceus* (Fisch.), *Mentha piperita* L., *Origanum vulgare* L., *Symphytum officinale* L., *Tanacetum parthenium* (L.) Schultz-Bip. and *Ulmus fulva* Michx.

The majority of the plants had antiviral and bacteriocidal activity against common pathogens, immunostimulation ability, antioxidant activity, and anti-inflammatory effects.

Keywords: British Columbia, pets, infectious tracheobronchitis, parvovirus, medicinal plants

1. Introduction

This chapter deals with some of the bacterial and viral conditions in pets that were treated with medicinal plants in British Columbia. Previous ethnoveterinary research has looked at anti-viral activity. For example six of the 17 plant extracts used by the Hausa and other tribes of Northern Nigeria for symptoms probably indicative of viral illness had antiviral activity (Kudi and Myint, 1999).

Infectious tracheobronchitis (ITB) or kennel cough is one of the conditions discussed in this chapter. It is an acute, highly contagious, global, respiratory disease in dogs affecting the larynx, trachea, bronchi, and occasionally the nasal mucosa and the lower respiratory tract. Dogs with the condition cough and show respiratory distress. Many agents play a role in ITB, such as canine parainfluenza virus, canine adenovirus, *Bordetella bronchiseptica*, mycoplasmas and *Streptococcus equi* subsp. *zooepidemicus* (Buonavoglia and Martella, 2007). Outbreaks of influenza A virus, initially misdiagnosed as ITB, were reported in the USA. New canine coronaviruses have been found in the respiratory tract of either symptomatic or asymptomatic dogs (Buonavoglia and Martella, 2007). Mammalian orthoreoviruses were found in dogs with pneumonia or enteritis, in association with either canine distemper virus or canine parvovirus type 2 (Buonavoglia and Martella, 2007).

Zarnke et al., 2004 conducted a serological suvey in 1,122 wolves in Alaska and the Yukon from 1984–2000. Antibody prevalence for canine hepatitis virus (ICH) was .84% for all areas. Area-specific prevalences of antibodies ranged from 12% to 70% for canine parvovirus (CPV), from 0% to 41% for canine distemper virus (CDV), and from 4% to 21% for *Francisella tularensis*.

The research participants claimed that 'dog show crud' mimics parvovirus but it gets worse if antibiotics are given. The signs are vomiting and diarrhoea. It is caused by an intestinal bacterium *Campylobacter jejuni* that is found in the soil on Vancouver Island. *Campylobacter upsaliensis* is a microorganism that is widespread on all continents and that is primarily isolated from the intestinal environment of dogs (Lentzsch et al., 2004). Its relevance as a pathogen that causes enteric diseases in animals is not clear, but it is recognized as a human pathogen.

McMyne et al., (1982) conduted serotyping of *Campylobacter jejuni* isolated from sporadic cases and outbreaks in the human population in British Columbia and found geographical differences. Ninety-six *Campylobacter upsaliensis* strains that originated from Australia, Canada, and Europe (Germany) and that were isolated from humans, dogs, and cats were serotyped (Lentzsch et al., 2004). Very few of the strains were isolated from cats and only *Campylobacter jejuni* from humans.

2. Materials and methods

Already presented.

3. Results

3.1 Treatment for an unknown infection

This particular unknown infection in a dog was treated with an herb that was said to acti like an antibiotic- *Usnea*. A tea was made with ½ cup *Usnea* to 2 cups of boiling water (dose used was 1 tsp/day strained tea for a 25 lb dog, twice a day for a month. For acute conditions a 1:1 tincture was made and 20 drops were given twice a day for two weeks).

An unknown infection in a cat was treated with an uva-ursi infusion (1 tsp of ground dry *Arctostaphylos uva-ursi* leaves in 1 cup of water). The 10-15 lb cat was given 2 tbsp of the strained infusion twice a day with food for three days. Other respondents used an uva-ursi tincture (30 to 60 drops in water four times daily for four days, not more).

Unknown infections in pets were also treated with a commercial extract of goldenseal (*Hydrastis canadensis*) and black cohosh (*Actaea racemosa*) (3 mg/lb). A homemade extract of black cohosh dried root was also used (10 – 25 mg/lb three times a day). Another treatment consisted of 2 tbsp each of powdered *Astragalus* (*Astragalus membranaceus*) and slippery elm bark (*Ulmus fulva*) with enough water to make a liquid that was given to the dog (40 to 45 lbs bodyweight) orally with a syringe.

3.2 Treatment for an unknown virus

Two dogs (11 lb and 3 lb) were losing weight and had to be forced to drink water and eat. They were also too weak to climb stairs or walk for long periods. Blood work of $250 revealed no cause and antibiotics only reduced the high fevers slightly. They had very foul breath. One dog (11 lb) was given 3 drops of echinamide (purchased Echinacea derived product) in 3 cc of water syringed into his mouth. The other dog (3 lbs) was given 2 drops in 2 cc water directly into the smaller dog's mouth. Both dogs were given water by syringe since they were not drinking. A purchased tincture of berries and flowers of hawthorn (*Crataegus oxycantha* was used as a general tonic. The crataegus tincture was made from crataegus bud only (gemmotherapy) (5 drops/3cc water (11 lb dog) and 3 drops/2cc water drops (3 lb dog) respectively, again in water and syringed into the mouth).

3.3 Treatment for dog show crud

Dog show crud is treated with 10 drops *Echinacea* and 10 drops purchased tincture of licorice root (*Glycyrrhiza glabra*) every three hours for four days (per 50 to 60 lb patient bodyweight). After recovery from the illness the dose is reduced to three times a day. Alternatively 10 drops purchased goldenseal (*Hydrastis canadensis*) root tincture is used. The pet was also given a broth of rice and barley. Twice a day the following was added to the diet: ¼ tsp slippery elm and Acidophilus. Alternatively 1 to 3 drops of Oregon grape root tincture (*Berberis aquifolium/ aquifolium*) was given (this was a 1:1 alcohol tincture).

3.4 Treatment for infectious tracheobronchitis

Dogs were given a strongly-brewed tea of mullein (*Verbascum thapsus*) for two weeks for infectious tracheobronchitis (¼ cup dried leaves to 1 cup of water, or a handful of fresh leaves to 1 cup of water). One tsp of the tea per 30lb bodyweight is put in the lip three times a day. The tea is given until all the symptoms are gone.

3.4.1. Case study of infectious tracheobronchitis

Patient: 7 month old female Labrador Retriever, 37 lbs.

The dog was given ¼ clove garlic per day (*Allium sativum*). Purchased capsules were used and coughing decreased significantly within 12 hours. During the participatory workshop the formula for a decoction using the same plants as in the purchased capsule was worked out. This consists of ¼ cup dried aerial parts of mullein (*Verbascum thapsus*), ¼ cup of coltsfoot (*Tussilago farfara*), ¼ cup of Oregon grape (*Berberis aquifolium*), and ¼ cup of marshmallow (*Althaea officinalis*) in 2 cups of water.

An alternative treatment consists of a tea made with 2 tbsp blossoms of red clover (*Trifolium pratense*), 1/3 cup chopped chickweed (*Stellaria media*), ¼ cup leaves of plantain (*Plantago major*) and 2 tbsp flowers of calendula (*Calendula officinalis*) per 10 to 15 lb patient bodyweight. Treatment is continued until the symptoms are gone.

3.5. Case study of parvo

The immune system of dogs with parvovirus was boosted with a tincture of goldenseal (*Hydrastis canadensis*) given orally (2 drops of tincture to 10 drops of water, per 25 lbs bodyweight three times daily). Additionally undiluted bleach was put on the stools for two weeks. The dogs' food had 1 tsp of the following herbs sprinkled on it every day: peppermint (*Mentha piperita*), comfrey (*Symphytum officinalis*), oregano (*Origanum* sp.) and feverfew (*Tanacetum parthenium*). A tsp of slippery elm bark powder (*Ulmus fulva*) was given to soothe the colon of the dogs. The dogs were also given 1 tsp brewers yeast for its nutritional properties and 1 drop per lb patient bodyweight of purchased *Astragalus* tincture. During the parvo outbreak one dog self medicated by eating 2 whole feverfew plants (*Tanacetum parthenium*). Feverfew is said to put a slippery coating on the toxins.

3.6. Treatment for an unknown virus

An owner's cats were not behaving normally. The owner assumed that a virus was present in the environment. The cats were given 2 or 3 drops of Echinacea (*Echinacea* spp.) tincture per 5 to 10 lbs bodyweight in the drinking water for three or four days. N.B. A strong dose of *Echinacea* will cause the cat to foam at the mouth. Dogs with an unknown virus can be given 20 drops of Echinacea (*Echinacea* spp.) tincture per 25 lbs bodyweight.

3.7. Treatment for colds and flu

For colds and flu teas or tinctures were made with any one of the following:

Garlic - (*Allium sativum*) or Scotch pine (*Pinus contorta*) needles and young bark.

Pets are also given 1 or 2 drops of tincture of Echinacea roots (*Echinacea angustifolia*, *Echinacea purpurea*, *Echinacea pallida*). *Echinacea* is not used for longer than eight weeks or together with anabolic steroids. Eucalyptus oil (1 – 2 drops per day) is given orally. Eucalyptus oil is always diluted in warm water before administration to a pet.

Oregano (*Origanum vulgaris*) tea is also used for colds but is not given during pregnancy. Teas made of yarrow, catnip (*Nepeta cataria*), sage (*Salvia officinalis*) or thyme (*Thymus vulgaris*) are also used. Pets are also given hyssop (*Hyssopus officinalis*) dried aerial parts as a tea or tincture.

3.8 Treatment for coughs

One small pet with coughs was given 1 tsp of purchased catnip tincture daily. Larger animals were given 2 tsp purchased tincture.

For coughs pets are given 1/3 chopped garlic clove (*Allium sativum*) or 2 mg garlic oil capsule. A typical dose is 1 clove per 40 – 50 lb patient bodyweight.

Owners are careful not to overdose with garlic. 5g/kg garlic is a toxic dose for cats.

For dry coughs the pet is given an infusion of marshmallow (*Althaea officinalis*) roots or a syrup made of the flowers. The infusion is made with ¼ cup dried powdered root in 6 cups of water (1 tbsp per 25 lbs of the pet's weight administered in the food or water until symptoms disappear).

Pets are also given a tea made of dill, fennel and catnip. The combination tea is made with 2 tbsp crushed dill (*Anethum graveolens*) seeds, leaves and flowers with 2 tbsp crushed fennel (*Foeniculum vulgare*) seeds, leaves, roots and 2 tbsp flowering tops of catnip (*Nepeta cataria*) with 3 cups of boiling water (1 tsp daily in food per 45 to 50 lb patient bodyweight). Fennel oil is not used since it is toxic. Other pets are given decoctions made with 1 tbsp of the following herbs: licorice root, marshmallow root, plantain leaves, thyme leaf. Decoctions are made with 3 cups of boiling water added to the herbs (1 tbsp daily per 25 lb patient bodyweight in the food or water).

An alternative tea can be made with 1 tsp fresh daisy (*Bellis perennis*) flowers in 1 cup of boiling water (1 tbsp strained liquid per 25 lbs bodyweight daily in the drinking water). Scotch pine (*Pinus contorta*) needles and young bark are also used to make an infusion (1 tbsp infusion daily in water or 1 - 2 drops per 50 – 55 lb patient bodyweight daily for a commercial tincture).

For chronic coughs pets are given a decoction of ¼ cup seeds, leaves and roots of plantain (*Plantago major, P. minor, P. lanceolata*) with ¼ cup flowers and leaves of mullein (*Verbascum thapsus*) in 3 cups of boiling water. The dose used is 1 tbsp per 25 lbs bodyweight in water until symptoms disappear. Wet coughs were treated with ½ - 1 tsp finely chopped ginger roots (*Zingiber officinalis*) (per 50 – 60 lb patient bodyweight) added to the food daily for 1 week.

4. Discussion

The non-experimental validation of the plants is presented in Table 24, in alphabetical order of the plants' scientific names. This validation process was started during the data collection phase and continued thereafter. Medicinal plant compounds with antiviral activity include terpenes, lignans, steroidal glycosides, thiosulfinates, proanthocyanidins and proteins (Chiang et al., 2002), many of the compounds are represented in the Table. Many of the plants have several biologically active compounds, for example *Plantago major* has five classes of biologically active compounds. These are: a benzoic compound (vanillic acid), flavonoids (baicalein, baicalin, luteolin), an iridoid glycoside (aucubin), phenolic compounds (caffeic acid, chlorogenic acid, ferulic acid, p-coumaric acid) and triterpenes (oleanolic acid, ursolic acid). The compounds ferulic acid and caffeic acid are active against herpes simplex virus 2 (HSV-2) *in vitro* and an aqueous extract of *Plantago major* has limited activity against herpes virus (Chiang et al., 2002). It is important to find biological activity in aqueous extracts because medicinal plants are often administered as teas. Triterpenoid glycosides have been isolated from black cohosh, and they exhibit anti-HIV activity while actaealactone is a lignan from the plant with biological activity (Nuntanakorn et al., 2006). Allitridin (diallyl trisulfide), one active compound of *Allium sativum* (garlic), can inhibit the expression of immediate-early antigens and viral proliferation of human cytomegalovirus (HCMV) *in vitro* (Liu et al., 2004).

5. Conclusion

Wang et al., (2006) claim that herbs act as anti-influenza agents in two ways:

inactivating or restraining the virus directly or have indirect activity by inducing interferon or regulating immune function. Anti-viral activity is typically linked to polyphenols, flavonoids, saponins, glucosides and alkaloids such as those found in *Mentha* species and *Zingiber* species (Wang et al., 2006). The second group of herbs categroised by Wang et al. (2006) are used to enhance or regulate immune function. They accomplish this by promoting phagocytosis by the reticuloendothelial system to enhance the immune function of the cell. Secondly, they induce interferons. Third, they enhance macrophage activation. *Astragalus membranaceus* is one of the plants with immunostimulant activity. *Berberis vulgaris* is immunosuppressive and *Echinacea purpurea* has the potential for enhancement of humoral immune responses as well as innate immune responses.

References

Alawa, J.P., Jokthan, G.E., Akut, K. 2002. Ethnoveterinary medical practice for ruminants in the subhumid zone of northern Nigeria. Prev Vet Med 54, 79 - 90.

Allan, P., Bilkei, G. 2005. Oregano improves reproductive performance of sows. Theriogenology. 63, 716-21.

Anon, 2000. Berberine monograph. Alternative Medicine Review 5, 175 – 177.

Anon, 2006. Effects of melatonin and motherwort tincture on the emotional state and visual functions in anxious subjects. Eksp Klin Farmakol. 69,17-9. Article in Russian.

Avato, P., Vitali, C., Mongelli, P., Tava, A. 1997. Antimicrobial activity of polyacetylenes from *Bellis perennis* and their synthetic derivatives. Planta Med. 63, 503-7.

Beaux, D., Fleurentin, J., Mortier, F. 1999. Effect of extracts of *Orthosiphon stamineus* Benth, *Hieracium pilosella* L., *Sambucus nigra* L. and *Arctostaphylos uva-ursi* (L.) Spreng. in rats. Phytother Res. 13, 222-5.

Blumenthal, M. 2000. Interactions Between Herbs and Conventional Drugs: Introductory Considerations. In: Herbs—everyday reference for health professionals. Ottawa: Canadian Pharmacists Association and Canadian Medical Association.

Bonjar, G.H. 2004. Inhibition of Clotrimazole-resistant *Candida albicans* by plants used in Iranian folkloric medicine. Fitoterapia 75,74-6.

Bouidida, el H., Alaoui, K., Cherrah, Y., Fkih-Tetouani, S., Idrissi, AI. 2006. Acute toxicity and analgesic activity of the global extracts of *Nepeta atlantica* Ball and *Nepeta tuberosa* L. ssp. reticulata (Desf.) Maire. Therapie. 61,447-52. Article in French.

Buonavoglia C, Martella V. 2007. Canine respiratory viruses. Vet Res. 38, 355-73.

Cai, Y., Luo, Q., Sun, M., Corke, H. 2004. Antioxidant activity and phenolic compounds of 112 traditional Chinese medicinal plants associated with anticancer. Life Sciences 74, 2157–2184.

Calixto, J.B., Beirith, A., Ferreira, J., Santos, A.R., Filho, V.C., Yunes, R.A. 2000. Naturally occurring antinociceptive substances from plants. Phytother Res. 14, 401-18.

Chadwick, L.R., Pauli, G.F., Farnsworth, N.R. 2006. The pharmacognosy of *Humulus lupulus* L. (hops) with an emphasis on estrogenic properties. Phytomedicine 13, 119-31.

Chiang, L.C., Chiang, W., Chang, M.Y., Ng, L.T., Lin, C.C. 2002. Antiviral activity of *Plantago major* extracts and related compounds *in vitro*. Antiviral Res 55, 53-62.

Chiang, L.C., Chiang, W., Chang, M.Y., Lin, C.C. 2003. *In vitro* cytotoxic, antiviral and immunomodulatory effects of *Plantago major* and *Plantago asiatica*. Am J Chin Med. 31, 225-34.

Cordova, C.A., Siqueira, I.R., Netto, C.A., Yunes, R.A., Volpato, A.M., Cechinel Filho, V., Curi-Pedrosa, R., Creczynski-Pasa, T.B. 2002. Protective properties of butanolic extract of the

Calendula officinalis L. (marigold) against lipid peroxidation of rat liver microsomes and action as free radical scavenger. Redox Rep. 7, 95-102.

Cowan, M.M. 1999. Plant products as antimicrobial agents. Clinical Microbiology Reveiws, 564–582.

Craig, W.J. 1999. Health-promoting properties of common herbs. Am J Clin Nutr. 70 (suppl), 491S–9S.

Denyer, C..V., Jackson, P., Loakes, D.M. 1994. Isolation of antirhinoviral sesquiterpenes from ginger (*Zingiber officinale*). J Nat Prod 57, 658-662.

Duke, J.A.1990. Promising phytomedicinals. In: J. Janick and J.E. Simon (eds.), Advances in new crops. Timber Press, Portland, OR.

Eberhardt, T.L., Young, R.A. 1996. Assessment of the anti-HIV activity of a pine cone isolate. Planta Med. 62, 63-5.

Freier, D.O., Wright, K., Klein, K., Voll, D., Dabiri, K., Cosulich, K., George, R. 2003. Enhancement of the humoral immune response by *Echinacea purpurea* in female Swiss mice. Immunopharmacol Immunotoxicol. 25, 551-60.

Gollapudi, S., Sharma, H.A., Aggarwal, S., Byers, L.D., Ensley, H.E., Gupta, S. 1995. Isolation of a previously unidentified polysaccharide (MAR-10) from *Hyssop officinalis* that exhibits strong activity against human immunodeficiency virus type 1. *Biochemical and Biophysical Research Communications* 210, 145-51.

Gomez-Flores, R., Calderon, C.L., Scheibel, L.W., Tamez-Guerra, P., Rodrigues-Padilla, C., Tames-Guerra, R., Weber, R.J. 2000. Immunoenhancing properties of *Plantago major* leaf extract. Phytother Res 14, 617-22.

Guil, J.L., Rodriguez-Garcia, I., Torija, E. 1997. Nutritional and toxic factors in selected wild edible plants. Plant Foods Hum Nutr. 51, 99-107.

Hersch-Martinez, P., Leanos-Miranda, B.E., Solorzano-Santos, F. 2005 Antibacterial effects of commercial essential oils over locally prevalent pathogenic strains in Mexico. Fitoterapia 76, 453-7.

Hubbert, M., Sievers, H., Lehnfeld, R., Kehrl, W. 2006. Efficacy and tolerability of a spray with *Salvia officinalis* in the treatment of acute pharyngitis - a randomised, double-blind, placebo-controlled study with adaptive design and interim analysis. Eur J Med Res. 11, 20-6.

Hussein, G., Miyashiro, H., Nakamura, N., Hattori, M., Kakiuchi, N., Shimotohno, K. 2000. Inhibitory effects of Sudanese medicinal plant extracts on Hepatitis C Virus (HCV) protease. Phytotherapy Research 14, 510 – 516.

Iauk, L., Costanzo, R., Caccamo, F., Rapisarda, A., Musumeci, R., Milazzo, I., Blandino, G. 2006. Activity of *Berberis aetnensis* root extracts on Candida strains. Fitoterapia. 78(2):159-61.

Imanishi, N., Andoh, T., Mantani, N., Sakai, S., Terasawa, K., Shimada, Y., Sato, M., Katada,Y., Ueda, K., Ochiai, H. 2006. Macrophage-mediated inhibitory effect of *Zingiber officinale* Rosc, a traditional oriental herbal medicine, on the growth of influenza A/Aichi/2/68 virus. Am J Chin Med. 34,157-69.

Jain, N.K., Kulkarni, S.K. 1999. Antinociceptive and anti-inflammatory effects of *Tanacetum parthenium* L. extract in mice and rats. J Ethnopharmacol. 68,251-9.

Jassim, S.A.A., Naji, M.A. 2003. Novel antiviral agents: a medicinal plant perspective. Journal of Applied Microbiology 95, 412–427.

Kemmerich, B., Eberhardt, R., Stammer, H. 2006. Efficacy and tolerability of a fluid extract combination of thyme herb and ivy leaves and matched placebo in adults suffering from acute bronchitis with productive cough. A prospective, double-blind, placebo-controlled clinical trial. Arzneimittelforschung. 56, 652-60.

Kim, M.R., Lee, J.Y., Lee, H.H., Aryal, D.K., Kim, Y.G., Kim, S.K., Woo, E.R., Kang, K.W. 2006. Antioxidative effects of quercetin-glycosides isolated from the flower buds of *Tussilago farfara* L. Food Chem Toxicol. 44, 1299-307.

Krivenko, V.V., Potebnia, G.P., Loiko, V.V. 1989. Experience in treating digestive organ diseases with medicinal plants. Vrach Delo 3,76-8. Article in Russian.

Kudi, A.C., and Myint, S.H. 1999. Antiviral activity of some Nigerian medicinal plant extracts. J Ethnopharmacol 68, 289 – 294.

Langmead, L., Dawson, C., Hawkins, C., Banna, N., Loo, S., Rampton, D.S. 2002. Antioxidant effects of herbal therapies used by patients with inflammatory bowel disease: an *in vitro* study. Aliment Pharmacol Ther. 16,197-205.

Lentzsch, P., Rieksneuwohner, B., Wieler, L.H., Hotzel, H., Moser, I. 2004. High-resolution genotyping of *Campylobacter upsaliensis* strains originating from three continents. J Clin Microbiol.42, 3441-8.

Li, Y.P., Wang, Y.M. 1988. Evaluation of tussilagone: a cardiovascular-respiratory stimulant isolated from Chinese herbal medicine. Gen Pharmacol. 19,261-3.

Liu ZF, Fang F, Dong YS, Li G, Zhen H. 2004. Experimental study on the prevention and treatment of murine cytomegalovirus hepatitis by using allitridin. Antiviral Res. 61, 125-8.

Lopez, P., Sanchez, C., Batlle, R., Nerin, C. 2005. Solid- and vapor-phase antimicrobial activities of six essential oils: susceptibility of selected foodborne bacterial and fungal strains. Journal of Agricultural and Food Chemistry 53, 6939–6946.

Lu, X.Q., Tang, F.D., Wang, Y., Zhao, T., Bian, R.L. 2004. Effect of *Eucalyptus globulus* oil on lipopolysaccharide-induced chronic bronchitis and mucin hypersecretion in rats. Zhongguo Zhong Yao Za Zhi 29,168-71. Article in Chinese.

Luo, C.N., Lin, X., Li, W.K., Pu, F., Wang, L.W., Xie, S.S., Xiao, P.G. 1998. Effect of berbamine on T-cell mediated immunity and the prevention of rejection on skin transplants in mice. J Ethnopharmacol. 59, 211-5.

Mathias, E. 2004. Ethnoveterinary medicine: Harnessing its potential. Vet Bull 74 , 27N – 37N.

McKay, D.L., Blumberg, J.B. 2006. A review of the bioactivity and potential health benefits of peppermint tea (*Mentha piperita* L.). Phytother. Res. 20, 619–633.

McMyne, P.M., Penner, J.L., Mathias, R.G., Black, W.A., Hennessy, J.N. 1982. Serotyping of *Campylobacter jejuni* isolated from sporadic cases and outbreaks in British Columbia. J Clin Microbiol. 16, 281-5.

Miyazaki, H., Matsuura, H., Yanagiya, C., Mizutani, J., Tsuji, M., Ishihara, C. 2003. Inhibitory effects of hyssop (*Hyssopus officinalis*) extracts on intestinal alpha-glucosidase activity and postprandial hyperglycemia. *Journal of Nutritional Science and Vitaminology* (Tokyo) 49 (5): 346-9.

Nosal'ova, G., Strapkova, A., Kardosova, A., Capek, P., Zathurecky, L., Bukovska, E. 1992. Antitussive action of extracts and polysaccharides of marsh mallow (*Althaea officinalis* L., var. robusta). Pharmazie. 47, 224-6. Article in German.

O'Neill, W., McKee, S., Clarke, A.F. 2002. Immunological and haematinic consequences of feeding a standardised Echinacea (*Echinacea angustifolia*) extract to healthy horses. Equine Vet J. 34, 222-7.

Nuntanakorn, P., Jiang, B., Einbond, L.S., Yang, H., Kronenberg, F., Weinstein, I.B., Kennelly, E.J. 2006. Polyphenolic Constituents of *Actaea racemosa*. J. Nat. Prod. 69, 314-318.

Pereira, R.S., Sumita, T.C., Furlan, M.R., Jorge, A.O., Ueno, M. 2004. Antibacterial activity of essential oils on microorganisms isolated from urinary tract infection. Rev Saude Publica 38,326-8. Article in Portuguese.

Rehman, J., Dillow, J.M., Carter, S.M., Chou, J., Le, B., Maisel, A.S. 1999. Increased production of antigen-specific immunoglobulins G and M following *in vivo* treatment with the medicinal plants *Echinacea angustifolia* and *Hydrastis canadensis*. Immunol Lett. 68, 391-5.

Sarrell, E.M., Cohen, H.A., Kahan, E. 2003 Naturopathic treatment for ear pain in children. Pediatrics 111(5 Pt 1), e574-9.

Shimizu, M., Shiota, S., Mizushima, T., Ito, H., Hatano, T., Yoshida, T., Tsuchiya, T. 2001. Marked potentiation of activity of beta-lactams against methicillin-resistant *Staphylococcus aureus* by corilagin. Antimicrob Agents Chemother 45, 3198-201.

Sauter, C., Wolfensberger, C. 1989. Anticancer activities as well as antiviral and virus-enhancing properties of aqueous fruit extracts from fifty-six European plant species. Eur J Cancer Clin Oncol 25, 987-990.

Silva, J., Abebe, W., Sousa, S.M., Duarte, V.G., Machado, M.I., Matos, F.J. 2003. Analgesic and anti-inflammatory effects of essential oils of *Eucalyptus*. J Ethnopharmacol. 89,277-83.

Stavri, M., Gibbons, S. 2005. The antimycobacterial constituents of dill (*Anethum graveolens*). Phytother Res. 19, 938-41.

Tunón, H., Olavsdotter, C., Bohlin, L. 1995. Evaluation of anti-inflammatory activity of some Swedish medicinal plants. Inhibition of prostaglandin biosynthesis andPAF-induced exocytosis. Journal of Ethnopharmacology 48: 61-76.

Turkera, U., Camper, N.D. 2002. Biological activity of common mullein, a medicinal plant. Journal of Ethnopharmacology 82, 117 – 125.

Ukiya, M., Akihisa, T., Yasukawa, K., Tokuda, H., Suzuki, T., Kimura, Y. 2006. Anti-Inflammatory, anti-tumor-promoting, and cytotoxic activities of constituents of marigold (*Calendula officinalis*) flowers. J. Nat. Prod. 69, 1692 – 1696.

Vermani, K., Garg, S., 2002. Herbal medicines for sexually transmitted diseases and AIDS. Journal of Ethnopharmacology 80, 49-66.

Vigo, E., Cepeda, A., Gualillo, O., Perez-Fernandez, R. 2004. *In-vitro* anti-inflammatory effect of *Eucalyptus globulus* and *Thymus vulgaris*: nitric oxide inhibition in J774A.1 murine macrophages. J Pharm Pharmacol. 56, 257-63.

Vijayan, P., Raghu, C., Ashok, G., Dhanaraj, S.A., Suresh, B. 2004. Antiviral activity of medicinal plants of Nilgiris. Indian Journal of Medical Research 120, 24 – 29.

Wang, S., Panter, K.E., Gardner, D.R., Evans, R.C., Bunch, T.D. 2004. Efects of the pine needle abortifacient, isocupressic acid, on bovine oocyte maturation and preimplantation embryo development. Anim Reprod Sci. 81, 237-44.

Wang, X., Jia, W., Aihua Zhao, A., Wang, X. 2006. Anti-influenza agents from plants and Traditional Chinese Medicine. Phytother. Res. 20, 335–341.

Weber, N.D., Anderson, D.O., North, J.A., Murray, B.K., Lawson, L.D., Hughes, B.G. 1992. *In vitro* virucidal effects of *Allium sativum* (garlic) extract and compounds. Planta Medica 58, 417-423.

Widyarini, S., Spinks, N., Husband, A.J., Reeve, V.E. 2001. Isoflavonoid compounds from red clover (*Trifolium pratense*) protect from inflammation and immune suppression induced by UV radiation. Photochem Photobiol. 74, 465-70.

Williams, C.A., Hoult, J.R., Harborne, J.B., Greenham, J., Eagles, J. 1995. A biologically active lipophilic flavonol from *Tanacetum parthenium*. Phytochemistry 38, 267-70.

Wynn, S.G., Marsden, S.A. 2003. Manual of Natural Veterinary Medicine: Science and Tradition. Mosby: St Louis.

Yao, M., Ritchie, H.E., Brown-Woodman, P.D. 2005. A reproductive screening test of goldenseal. Birth Defects Res B Dev Reprod Toxicol. 74, 99-404.

Youn, H.J., Noh, J.W., 2001. Screening of the anticoccidial effects of herb extracts against *Eimeria tenella*. Vet Parasitol. 96, 257-63.

Zarnke, R.L., Ver Hoef, J.M., DeLong, R.A. 2004. Serologic survey for selected disease agents in wolves (*Canis lupus*) from Alaska and the Yukon Territory, 1984-2000. J Wildl Dis. 40, 632-8.

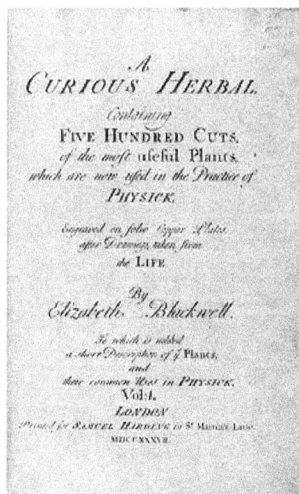

Illustration from Elizabeth Blackwell's *A Curious Herbal*

TABLE 21. TREATMENT FOR AN UNKNOWN INFECTION IN PETS THOUGHT TO BE TREATABLE WITH AN ANTIBIOTIC

Scientific name	Common name	Plant part used
Arctostaphylos uva-ursi (L.) Spreng. (Ericaceae)	uva-ursi	Leaves
Actaea racemosa L. var. *racemosa* (Ranunculaceae)	black cohosh	Root
Astragalus membranaceus (Fisch.) (Fabaceae)	astragalus	
Hydrastis canadensis L. (Ranunculaceae)	goldenseal	
Ulmus fulva Michx. (Ulmaceae)	slippery elm	Bark
Usnea longissima Ach. (Parmeliaceae)	usnea	

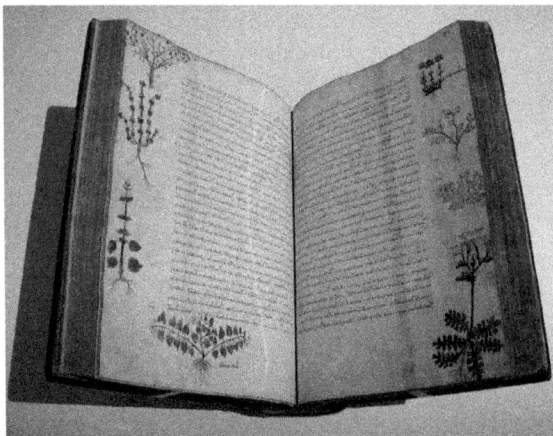

Dioscorides De Materia Medica Byzantium 15th century.jpg

TABLE 22. ETHNOVETERINARY REMEDIES USED IN BRITISH COLUMBIA FOR PETS WITH VIRAL INFECTIONS

Scientific name	Common name	Plant part used	Use
Allium sativum L. (Alliaceae)	garlic	clove	Case study of infectious tracheobronchitis
Althaea officinalis L. (Malvaceae)	marshmallow		Case study of infectious tracheobronchitis
Astragalus membranaceus (Fisch.) (Fabaceae)	astragalus		parvo case study
Berberis aquifolium Pursh./ *Mahonia aquifolium* (Berberidaceae)	Oregon grape		Case study of infectious tracheobronchitis
Calendula officinalis L. (Asteraceae)	calendula		infectious tracheobronchitis
Crataegus oxycantha (Rosaceae)	hawthorn	Buds or berries & flowers	case study unknown virus (2 dogs)
Echinacea purpurea (L.) Moench (Asteraceae)	echinacea		case study unknown virus (2 dogs), dog show crud
Glycyrrhiza glabra L. (Fabaceae)	licorice	root	dog show crud
Hydrastis canadensis L. (Ranunculaceae)	goldenseal		dog show crud, parvo case study
Mahonia nervosa (Pursh) Nutt (Berberidaceae)	Oregon grape	root	dog show crud
Mentha piperita L. (Lamiaceae)	peppermint		parvo case study
Origanum vulgare L. (Labiatae)	oregano		parvo case study
Plantago major L. (Plantaginaceae)	plantain		infectious tracheobronchitis
Stellaria media (L.) Cyrill. (Caryophyllaceae)	chickweed	aerial parts	infectious tracheobronchitis
Symphytum officinale L. (Boraginaceae)	comfrey		parvo case study
Tanacetum parthenium (L.) Schultz-Bip. (Asteraceae)	feverfew	aerial parts	parvo case study – self medication
Trifolium pratense L. (Fabaceae)	red clover	flowers	infectious tracheobronchitis
Tussilago farfara L.	coltsfoot		Case study of infectious

(Asteraceae)			tracheobronchitis
Ulmus fulva Michx. (Ulmaceae)	Slippery elm	bark	parvo case study- colon health, dog show crud
Verbascum thapsus L. (Scrophulariaceae)	mullein	aerial parts	Case study of infectious tracheobronchitis

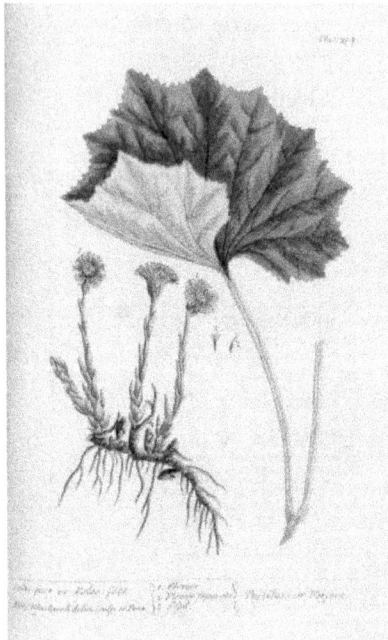

Illustration from Elizabeth Blackwell's *A Curious Herbal*

TABLE 23. ETHNOVETERINARY TREATMENTS FOR RESPIRATORY CONDITIONS IN PETS IN BC

Scientific name	Common name	Plant part used	Use
Achillea millefolium L. (Asteraceae)	yarrow	aerial parts, flowers	colds & flu
Allium sativum L. (Alliaceae)	garlic	clove	coughs, colds and flu
Althaea officinalis L. (Malvaceae)	marshmallow	roots, flowers	dry coughs, coughs
Anethum graveolens L. (Apiaceae)	dill	seeds, leaves & flowers	coughs
Bellis perennis L. (Asteraceae)	daisy	flowers	coughs
Echinacea purpurea (L.) Moench (Asteraceae)	Echinacea	root	colds & flu
Eucalyptus globules Labill. (Myrtaceae)	eucalyptus	leaf	colds & flu
Foeniculum vulgare Mill. (Umbelliferae)	fennel	seeds, leaves, roots	coughs
Glycyrrhiza glabra L. (Fabaceae)	licorice	root	coughs
Hyssopus officinalis L. (Lamiaceae)	hyssop	aerial parts	colds & flu
Nepeta cataria L. (Lamiaceae)	catnip	flowering tops	colds & flu, coughs
Origanum vulgare L. (Labiatae)	oregano	aerial parts	colds & flu
Pinus contorta (Pinaceae)	Scotch pine	needles & young bark	coughs, colds and flu
Plantago lanceolata L. (Plantaginaceae)	plantain	seeds, leaves, roots	chronic coughs
Plantago major L. (Plantaginaceae)	plantain	leaves	coughs
Salvia officinalis L. (Lamiaceae)	sage	leaf	colds & flu
Thymus vulgaris L. (Lamiaceae)	thyme	aerial parts	colds & flu, coughs
Verbascum thapsus L. (Scrophulariaceae)	mullein	flowers & leaves	chronic coughs
Zingiber officinalis Roscoe (Zingiberaceae)	ginger	roots	wet coughs

TABLE 24. NON-EXPERIMENTAL VALIDATION OF PLANTS USED FOR PETS IN BRITISH COLUMBIA

Medicinal plant	Validation information	Reference
Achillea millefolium	*Achillea millefolium* is used for colds and flu in our study and has antiinflammatory activity. Quercetagetin has anti-HIV activity.	Tunón et al., 1995; Vermani and Garg, 2002
Actaea racemosa	*Actaea racemosa* is used in place of an antibiotic by pet owners. More than 40 triterpenoid glycosides are found in black cohosh, with various biological activities including anti-HIV activity, and inhibitory effects on catecholamine secretion. Thirteen polyphenolic derivatives were isolated from the rhizomes and roots of black cohosh, including hydroxycinnamic acid derivatives (e.g., caffeic acid, ferulic acid, and isoferulic acid), fukiic acid ester derivatives, and piscidic acid ester derivatives. Black cohosh compounds are reported to have anti-inflammatory, and antioxidant activities and exhibit inhibitory effects on the enzymatic activities of R-amylase, carboxypeptidase A, and collagenase.	Nuntanakorn Et al., 2006
Allium sativum	Garlic was used for respiratory problems in our study. Allicin inhibits a wide variety of bacteria, molds, yeasts (including Candida), and viruses, including influenza viruses. Garlic shows an immunopotentiating effect by stimulating natural killer cell activity. Allicin and ajoene are active compounds.	Weber etal., 1992; Craig, 2007
Althaea officinalis	*Althaea officinalis* was used to treat coughs in pets. The complex extract and the polysaccharide isolated from the roots of marshmallow were tested for antitussive activity in unanaesthetized cats of both sexes. The polysaccharide in a dose of 50 mg/kg b.w. was as effective in inhibition of the cough reflex as Sirupus Althaeae in a dose of 1000 mg/kg b.w. and more effective than prenoxdiazine in a dose of 30 mg/kg b.w. However, the cough-suppressing effect of the polysaccharide was lower than that of dropropizine. The extract was less effective than the polysaccharide. Marshmallow has been used as an expectorant to treat a variety of upper respiratory problems and gastric ulcers in humans. Absorption of other drugs taken simultaneously with marshmallow (*Althea officinalis*) may be delayed because of its high mucilage content.	Nosal'ova et al., 1992; Wynn and Marsden, 2003; Blumenthal, 2000
Anethum	In our research, dill was used to treat coughs. The	Stavri and

graveolens	monoterpene carvone is a major constituent (50%–60%) of the essential oil and has a sedative effect. Falcarindiol from the whole herb of *Anethum graveolens* had minimum inhibitory concentration (MIC) values in the range 2–4 µg/mL against mycobacteria (*Mycobacterium fortuitum*, *Mycobacterium phlei*, *Mycobacterium aurum* and *Mycobacterium smegmatis*). Plant compounds oxypeucedanin and oxypeucedanin hydrate showed moderate anti-mycobacterial activity against the same mycobacteria with MIC values in the range 32–128 µg/mL. Dill has many compounds with antiviral activity usch as eugenol and caffeic acid.	Gibbons, 2005; Lopez et al., 2005; Duke, 1990
Arctostaphylos uva-ursi	*Arctostaphylos uva-ursi* was used as an antibiotic replacement in our study. An extract of *Arctostaphylos uva-ursi* significantly reduced the MICs of beta-lactam antibiotics, such as oxacillin and cefmetazole, against methicillin-resistant *Staphylococcus aureus*. The active compound, corilagin, showed a synergistic bactericidal action when added to the growth medium in combination with oxacillin. This herb should not be administered with any substances that cause acidic urine, such as ascorbic acid and ammonium chloride, as it will reduce the antibacterial effect.	Beaux et al., 1999; Shimizu et al., 2001; Blumenthal, 2000
Astragalus membranaceus	*Astragalus membranaceus* was used as an antibiotic replacement in our study and in the case study on parvovirus. *Astragalus membranaceus* could be used for the treatment for malignant tumors. Astragalus root increases the immune-stimulating effects of interleukin-2 and acyclovir but may be incompatible with immunosuppressive drugs (e.g., cyclosporine, azathioprine and methotrexate). *Astragalus mongholicus* has antiviral activity. Yiqi Qingwen Jiedu Heji (a formula that includes *Astragalus membranaceus* can dampen the expression of pro-inflammatory cytokines thus alleviating inflammatory injury.	Zhao, 1993; Blumenthal, 2000; Wang et al., 2006
Bellis perennis	Daisies were one of the many plants used for coughs. Essential oils from the aerial organs of *Bellis perennis* L., contain polyacetylenes. Only deca-4,6-diynoic acid and deca-4,6-diyne-1,10-dioic acid showed antimicrobial activity against Gram-positive and Gram-negative bacteria, respectively.	Avato et al., 1997
Berberis vulgaris/ Mahonia nervosa	*Berberis vulgaris* was used for infectious tracheobronchitis. The pharmacologic actions of the alkaloid berberine include inhibition of bacterial enterotoxin formation, inhibition of intestinal fluid accumulation and ion secretion, reduction of	Anon, 2000; Iauk et al., 2006

	inflammation, platelet aggregation inhibition, platelet count elevation in certain types of thrombocytopenia and stimulation of bile and bilirubin secretion. It has a significant leukogenic effect, and is immunosuppressive. Antimicrobial activity is found in *Berberis heterophylla* and *B. aetnensis* the active compounds are berberine and berbamine, alkaloidal constituents of *Berberis* spp.	
Calendula officinalis	*Calendula officinalis* has many pharmacological properties and was used in our study to treat infectious tracheobronchitis. It is used for pain and also as a bactericide, antiseptic and anti-inflammatory. The butanolic fraction of *C. officinalis* possesses a significant free radical scavenging and antioxidant activity and the proposed therapeutic efficacy of this plant could be attributed to these properties. Chronic hyposecretory gastritis, chronic hepatocholecystitis and angiocholitis were treated with a herbal complex which included *Achillea millefolium*, *Urtica dioica*, *Cichorium* (aboveground part), *Polygonum*, *Matricaria chamomilla* (flowers), *Helichrysum arenarium*, *Calendula* (flowers), corn stigmas, *Humulus lupulus* (racemes). *Calendula* extracts of marigold show anti-HIV activities. Triterpene fatty acid esters show anti-inflammatory and antiedematous activities.4	Cordova et al. 2002; Klouchek-Popova et al. 2002; Krivenko et al.,1989
Crataegus oxycantha	Hawthorn was used to treat a suspected virus in dogs. Preparations made from flowers of *Crataegus* spp., with leaves (and fruits) may enhance the effects of cardiac glycosides and have been used with such drugs in German clinical medicine to reduce the risk of toxic effects. Hawthorn has increased barbiturate-induced sleeping times. *Crataegus pinnatifida* contains flavonoids (epicatechin, quercetin, vitexin, quercitrin), phenolic acids (chlorogenic acid). *Crataegus crus-galli* has activity against influenza.	Blumenthal, 2000
Echinacea purpurea	*Echinacea purpurea* was one of the many plants being used to treat colds and flu in our study. It has been investigated for its potential to enhance immune function, primarily through activation of innate immune responses. A time course study, using the time of SRBC immunization to mimic the onset of illness, examined the effects of 8 and 4 days of *Echinacea purpurea* treatment at 0.6 mL/kg/day. Only in the 4-day administration, with dosing beginning 1 hour after SRBC immunization, was there an observed enhancement of the antibody forming cell response. This supports the acute use of *Echinacea purpurea* as suggested by	Freier et al., 2002

	anecdotal reports, and demonstrates the potential for enhancement of humoral immune responses as well as innate immune responses.	
Eucalyptus globulus	Similarly to the use in humans, *Eucalyptus globulus* was used for colds in pets. The oil has an anti-inflammatory effect on chronic bronchitis induced by lipopolysaccharide in rats and an inhibitory effect on hypersecretion of airway mucins. Chemicals that alleviate swelling are derived from some essential oils such as clove, eucalyptus and pine. *Eucalyptus globulus* Labill. and *Thymus vulgaris* L. have been used in traditional medicine in the treatment of bronchitis, asthma and other respiratory diseases. *Eucalyptus citriodora*, *Eucalyptus tereticornis*, and *Eucalyptus globulus* possess central and peripheral analgesic effects as well as neutrophil-dependent and independent anti-inflammatory activities. The inhibition of net nitrogen oxide (NO) production by *Eucalyptus globulus* and *Thymus vulgaris* extracts may be due to their NO scavenging activity and/or their inhibitory effects on iNOS gene expression. Eucalyptus oil induces the liver enzyme system involved in detoxification, so the effects of other drugs can be weakened or shortened.	Lu et al., 2004; Darshan and Doreswamy, 2004; Silva et al., 2003; Vigo et al., 2004; Blumenthal, 2000
Foeniculum vulgare	Fennel was used to treat coughs in pets. *Foeniculum vulgare* contains phenolic acids (cinnamic acid, vanillic acid) and coumarins (6,7-dihydroxycoumarin). *Foeniculum vulgare* water extract had 33.1 ± 6.7 HCV-PR inhibition(%) against hepatitis C virus (HCV) protease (PR).	Cai et al., 2004; Hussein et al., 2000
Glycyrrhiza glabra	Coughs and dog show crud were treated with licorice. Stronger neominophagen C (SNMC) is a Japanese preparation that contains 0.2% glycyrrhizin, 0.1% cysteine, and 2% glyceine. SNMC has no antiviral properties; it acts as an anti-inflammatory or cytoprotective drug.	Dhiman and Chawla, 2005; Blumenthal, 2000
Hydrastis canadensis	Goldenseal (*Hydrastis canadensis*). had many uses in our study: dog show crud, parvo and as an antibiotic replacement. Botanical supplements containing goldenseal strongly inhibited CYP2D6 and CYP3A4/5 activity *in vivo* therefore serious adverse interactions may result from the concomitant ingestion of goldenseal supplements and drugs that are CYP2D6 and CYP3A4/5 substrates. Goldenseal contains the berberine alkaloid. Berberine extracts and decoctions have demonstrated significant antimicrobial activity against a variety of organisms including bacteria, viruses, fungi, protozoans,	Yao et al., 2005; Gurley et al., 2005; Blumenthal, 2000, Anon, 2000; Rehman et al., 1999

	helminths, and chlamydia. The predominant clinical uses of berberine include bacterial diarrhea, intestinal parasite infections, and ocular trachoma infections. Goldenseal can modulate the antigen-specific immune response, by enhancing the acute primary IgM response.	
Hyssopus officinalis	*Hyssopus officinalis* was used for colds and flu in our study and this use comes from the Cherokee. Efficacy studies with hyssop (*Hyssopus officinalis*) and hyssop oil have been conducted *in vitro*. Antimicrobial activity of hyssop is linked to polysaccharides, essential oil, caffeic acid, tannins, and specifically (-)-cis- and (-)-trans-3-pinanones (found in the oil of hyssop). Polysaccharides and crude extracts were active against HIV-type 1, HIV-3 and non-toxic to uninfected cells. Extracts suppress hyperglycemia. Terpenoids have antiviral activity. The dried plant is not known to have the toxin pinocamphone; however hyssop should not be used for long periods.	Gollapudi et al., 1995; Miyazaki et al., 2003; Cowan, 1999
Mentha piperita	*Mentha* was sprinked on the food of dogs with parvovirus. The salicylic acid content of peppermint tea is 0.2 mg/kg. Antiviral activity is evident in aqueous extracts of peppermint leaves towards influenza A, Newcastle disease virus, Herpes simplex virus (HSV) and Vaccinia virus in egg and cell-culture systems. An alcohol extract of *M. piperita* in combination with four other herbs (*Thymus serpyllum*, *Viscum album*, *Salvia officinalis* and *Glycyrrhiza glabra*) inhibited the reproduction of influenza viruses A/Gabrovo (H1N1), A/Hong Kong (H3N2) and A/PR/8 (H1N1) in tissue cultures and embryonated eggs. An aqueous extract of *M. piperita* was active against anti-human immunodeficiency virus-1 (HIV)-1 at 16 µg/mL in MT-4 cells. The major respiratory tract pathogens, including *Haemophilus influenzae*, *Streptococcus pneumoniae*, *Streptococcus pyogenes* and *Staphylococcus aureus*, were susceptible to peppermint oil and its components menthol and menthone, but not to 1,8-cineole. Menthol had an MIC range of 0.04–0.08% (w/v), with peppermint oil at 0.08–0.32%. Another respiratory tract pathogen, *Legionella pneumophila*, was also susceptible to peppermint.	McKay and Blumberg, 2006
Nepeta cataria	Catnip was used for respiratory problems in pets. Catnip (*Nepeta cataria*) (especially the volatile oil) may promote uterine contractions, so it should not be used during pregnancy. The global extracts of *Nepeta*	Bouidida et al., 2006; Calixto et al., 2000; Jassim and

	atlantica Ball and *Nepeta tuberosa* L. ssp. *reticulata* (Desf.) Maire contain iridoids and triterpines. The plants have analgesic activity. Nepetalactone, a lactone in *Nepeta casearea*, is the main antinociceptive component of this plant, and shows a specific opioid receptor subtype agonistic activity. 1,8-cineole, present in the essential oil of *Nepeta italica*, exhibited antinociception by interaction with the opioidergic pathway.*Nepeta coerulea, Nepeta nepetella* and *Nepeta tuberosa*, showed clear antiviral activity against DNA and RNA viruses (HSV-1 and VSV).	Naji, 2003
Origanum vulgare	Origanum vulgare was used for parvovirus and for respiratory problems in our study. In a field trial alternate farrowing groups were given diets containing 1000 ppm oregano (dried leaf and flower of Origanum vulgare, enriched with 500 g/kg of cold-pressed essential oils of O. vulgare) in prefarrowing and lactation diets. There were 801 oregano-treated sows, and 1809 untreated control sows. Sows fed oregano had lower annual sow mortality rate, lower sow culling rate during lactation, increased farrowing rate, increased number of liveborn piglets per litter, and decreased stillbirth rate and higher daily voluntary feed intake compared to non-treated sows. Alpha-pinene, Apigenin, ascorbic acid, beta-bisabolene and caffeic acid are some of the antiviral components in the plant.	Allan and Bilkei, 2005
Pinus contorta	*Pinus contorta* was used for respiratory problems in our study. Isocupressic acid (ICA) [15-hydroxylabda-8 (17), 13E-dien-19-oic acid], a labdane diterpene acid, isolated from ponderosa pine (*Pinus ponderosa*), lodgepole pine (*Pinus contorta*), common juniper (*Juniperus communis*) and Monterey cypress (*Cupressus macrocarpa*), induces abortion in pregnant cows when ingested primarily during the last trimester but needles do not compromise early reproductive processes in cattle. *Pinus nigra* Arnold seed cones contain a phenylpropanoid (i.c. lignin) component which may have anti-HIV-1 activity.	Wang et al., 2004; Eberhardt and Young, 1996
Plantago major	*Plantago* species were used for infectious tracheobronchitis and to treat respiratory problems. *Plantago major* Linn. and *P. asiatica* Linn. hot water extracts possess abroad-spectrum antileukemia, anticarcinoma and antiviral activities, as well as activities which modulate cell-mediated immunity.	Chiang et al., 2003; Gomez-Flores et al., 2000
Salvia officinalis	Pets were given sage to treat colds and flu. The efficacy and tolerability of a spray containing a *Salvia officinalis* fluid extract was tested against a placebo in the	Hubbert et al., 2006; Pereira et al., 2004

	treatment of patients with acute viral pharyngitis. In the first part of the study 122 patients were enrolled. The second part of the study included 164 patients. The treatment duration per patient was 3 days. A 15 % sage spray proved to be a safe treatment for patients with acute pharyngitis. Symptomatic relief occurred within the first two hours after first administration and was significantly superior to the placebo. *Salvia officinalis*, L. showed 100% efficiency against *Klebsiella* and *Enterobacter* species, 96% against *Escherichia coli*, 83% against *Proteus mirabilis*, and 75% against *Morganella morganii*.	
Stellaria media	Infectious tracheobronchitis was treated with *Stellaria media*.The carotenoid content of *Stellaria media* Villars was 4.2 mg/100 g The plant contains 12,936 ppm chlorine which is antiviral as is genistein and rutin.	Guil et al., 1997; Duke, 1990
Symphytum officinale	Comfrey was used for parvovirus in our study. The antiinflammatory activity of comfrey (*Symphytum officinale*) is linked to rosmarinic acid, which has antioxidant, antiviral, bactericidal and viricidal activities.	Duke, 1990
Tanacetum parthenium	*Tanacetum parthenium* was used for parvovirus in our study. A lipophilic flavonol called tanetin was found in the leaf, flower and seed of feverfew, *Tanacetum parthenium*. Tanetin could contribute to the anti-inflammatory properties of feverfew by inhibiting the generation of pro-inflammatory eicosanoids. Water soluble flavone glycosides were detected in the leaves. Oral administration of the feverfew (*Tanacetum parthenium*) extract led to significant antinociceptive and anti-inflammatory effects. Parthenolide (1, 2 mg/kg i.p.), one active constituent of the extract also produced antinociceptive and anti-inflammatory effects.	Williams et al., 1995; Jain and Kulkarni, 1999
Thymus vulgaris	Thyme oil (*Thymus vulgaris*) is used externally only for respiratory problems and the pet watched for sensitivities. Thyme (*Thymus vulgaris*) essential oil showed high and broad antibacterial activity against prevalent pathogenic bacteria. *In vitro* anticandidal activity of the methanol extracts of *Thymus vulgaris* was evaluated at a 20 mg/ml concentration against Clotrimazole-resistant *Candida albicans. Thymus vulgaris* had a MIC of 0.62 mg/ml. In a double-blind, placebo-controlled, multicentre Phase IV study 361 outpatients with acute bronchitis were randomly assigned to an 11-day treatment (5.4 ml three times daily) with either thyme-ivy combination syrup (Bronchipret Saft; N=182) or placebo syrup (N=179).	Hersch-Martinez et al., 2005; Bonjar, 2004; Kemmerich et al., 2006

	The mean reduction in coughing fits on days 7 to 9 relative to baseline was 68.7% under thyme-ivy combination compared to 47.6 % under placebo (p < 0.0001). Oral treatment of acute bronchitis with thyme-ivy combination for about 11 days was superior to placebo.	
Trifolium pratense	*Trifolium pratense* was used for infectious tracheobronchitis. Isoflavones have significant antioxidant, estrogenic and tyrosine kinase inhibitory activity. Genistein can provide protection from oxidative damage induced by UV radiation both *in vitro* and following dietary administration. Clover flowers have some antiviral compounds and the plant contains chlorogenic acid and genistein with antiviral activity.	Widyarini et al., 2001; Duke, 1990
Tussilago farfara	Infectious tracheobronchitis was treated with *Tussilago farfara*. In traditional Chinese herbal medicine Kuandong Hua/coltsfoot (*Tussilago farfara* L.) is used in the treatment of various respiratory conditions. An extract of the plant called Tussilagone (TUS) is a potent cardiovascular and respiratory stimulant. *Tussilago farfara* has antimicrobial activity, inhibitory activity against nitric oxide synthase and antagonistic activity on platelet-activating factor receptor.	Li and Wang, 1988; Kim et al., 2006
Ulmus fulva	*Ulmus fulva* was used as an antibiotic replacement for parvovirus, colon health and dog show crud .Herbal remedies used by patients for treatment of inflammatory bowel disease include slippery elm, fenugreek and devil's claw. One study examined the antioxidant effects of herbal remedies in cell-free oxidant-generating systems and inflamed human colorectal biopsies. All herbs, except fenugreek, scavenged superoxide dose-dependently. All materials tested scavenged peroxyl dose-dependently. Oxygen radical release from biopsies was reduced after incubation in all the tested herbs. All the herbal remedies had antioxidant effects. *Ulmus macrocarpa* seed and bark extract improved the survival rate of day-old broiler chicks infected with *Eimeria tenella*.	Langmead, 2002; Youn and Noh, 2001
Usnea longissima	*Usnea* was used as an antibiotic replacement in our study. *Usnea complanta* has been used for bacterial infections. It has antiviral activity	Vijayan et al., 2004
Verbascum thapsus	Chornic coughs and infectious tracheobronchitis were treated with *Verbascum thapsus*. It has traditionally been used for the treatment of inflammatory diseases, asthma, spasmodic coughs, diarrhea and other pulmonary problems. Mullein extracts prepared in water,	Turker and Camper, 2002

	ethanol and methanol had antibacterial activity (especially the water extract) on *Klebsiella pneumonia, Staphylococcus aureus, Staphylococcus epidermidis* and *Escherichia coli*.	
Verbascum thapsus	A study designed as a double-blind trial in an outpatient community clinic tested the Naturopathic Herbal Extract Ear Drops on 171 children who were aged 5 to 18 years and had otalgia and clinical findings associated with middle-ear infection were studied. Treatment was with Naturopathic Herbal Extract Ear Drops (NHED) or anaesthetic ear drops, with or without amoxicillin. The children were randomized to receive NHED (contents: *Allium sativum, Verbascum thapsus, Calendula flores, Hypericum perfoliatum*, lavender, and vitamin E in olive oil) 5 drops 3 times daily, alone (group A) or together with a topical aesthetic (amethocaine and phenazone in glycerin) 5 drops 3 times daily (group B), or oral amoxicillin 80 mg/kg/d (maximum 500 mg/dose) divided into 3 doses with either NHED 5 drops 3 times daily (group C) or topical anaesthetic 5 drops 3 times daily (group D). These herbal extracts had *in vitro* bacteriostatic and bacteriocidal activity against common pathogens, immunostimulation ability, antioxidant activity, and anti-inflammatory effects.	Sarrell et al., 2003
Zingiber officinalis	In our study ginger was used for wet coughs. The inhibitory effect of *Zingiber officinale* Rosc on the growth of influenza A/Aichi/2/68 (Aichi) virus was investigated in Madin-Darby canine kidney cells. Ginger itself had no inhibitory effect on the growth of influenza virus, but could exert its inhibitory effect via macrophage activation leading to production of TNF-alpha. Ginger has activity against rhinovirus.	Imanishi et al., 2006; Denyer et al., 1994

www.ingramcontent.com/pod-product-compliance
Lightning Source LLC
Chambersburg PA
CBHW051409200326
41520CB00023B/7169